ESSENTIAL SKILLS FOR A MEDICAL TEACHER

AN INTRODUCTION TO TEACHING AND LEARNING IN MEDICINE

Ronald M. Harden OBE MD FRCP(Glas) FRCPC FRCSEd
General Secretary, Association of Medical Education in Europe; Editor of
Medical Teacher; Former Professor of Medical Education, Director of the
Centre for Medical Education and Teaching Dean, University of Dundee, UK;
Professor of Medical Education Al-Imam University, Riyadh, Saudi Arabia.

Jennifer M. Laidlaw DipEdTech MMEd
Formerly Assistant Director, Education Development Unit, Scottish Council
for Postgraduate Medical and Dental Education at the University of Dundee,
Dundee, UK

Foreword by

Steven L. Kanter MD
Vice Dean, University of Pittsburgh School of Medicine, Pittsburgh, PA, USA

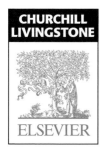

CHURCHILL
LIVINGSTONE

ELSEVIER

Edinburgh   London   New York   Oxford   Philadelphia   St Louis   Sydney   Toronto   2012

© 2012 Elsevier Ltd. All rights reserved.

ISBN 978-0-7020-4582-0

British Library Cataloguing in Publication Data
A catalogue record for this book is available from the British Library

Library of Congress Cataloging in Publication Data
A catalog record for this book is available from the Library of Congress

Notices
Knowledge and best practice in this field are constantly changing. As new research and experience broaden our understanding, changes in research methods, professional practices, or medical treatment may become necessary.

Practitioners and researchers must always rely on their own experience and knowledge in evaluating and using any information, methods, compounds, or experiments described herein. In using such information or methods they should be mindful of their own safety and the safety of others, including parties for whom they have a professional responsibility.

With respect to any drug or pharmaceutical products identified, readers are advised to check the most current information provided (i) on procedures featured or (ii) by the manufacturer of each product to be administered, to verify the recommended dose or formula, the method and duration of administration, and contraindications. It is the responsibility of practitioners, relying on their own experience and knowledge of their patients, to make diagnoses, to determine dosages and the best treatment for each individual patient, and to take all appropriate safety precautions.

To the fullest extent of the law, neither the Publisher nor the authors, contributors, or editors, assume any liability for any injury and/or damage to persons or property as a matter of products liability, negligence or otherwise, or from any use or operation of any methods, products, instructions, or ideas contained in the material herein.

ELSEVIER your source for books, journals and multimedia in the health sciences
www.elsevierhealth.com

Working together to grow libraries in developing countries
www.elsevier.com | www.bookaid.org | www.sabre.org
ELSEVIER   BOOK AID International   Sabre Foundation

The Publisher's policy is to use paper manufactured from sustainable forests

Printed in China

ESSENTIAL SKILLS
FOR A MEDICAL
TEACHER

To Jennifer

Love Dad.

Ronald Harden

Commissioning Editor: Laurence Hunter
Development Editor: Sally Davies
Project Manager: Lucy Boon
Designer/Design Direction: Greg Harris
Illustration Manager: Jennifer Rose

CONTENTS

CONTENTS

CONTENTS

FOREWORD

Telling someone how to be a better teacher is a most delicate matter. It ranks second in difficulty only to telling someone how to be a better parent.

Why is this so? Perhaps, in part, because many hold to the underlying, albeit false, assumption: "Once I was a student; therefore, I know how to teach."

Certainly, completing a course of study in a school of medicine provides important content expertise and invaluable experience that is necessary to be a good teacher of medical students. But it is not sufficient. There is a body of knowledge about teaching itself, instructional method, course and curriculum design, learning and assessment that should be mastered by anyone who plays a significant role in a medical education program.

In this book, Harden and Laidlaw present clear, concise and accessible information about each of these areas. They make the case that teaching is important, that one can learn how to be a better teacher, and that it is a most rewarding endeavor. They emphasize that it is essential for good teachers to learn the basics of teaching and that they must maintain a current knowledge of the latest developments in medical education.

The contents of this book offer candid, succinct and practical advice to an individual who is new to medical teaching, as well as to the more experienced teacher who has accepted new responsibilities for a seminar, a course or an entire program. Also, this book will be a valuable resource for those pursuing an advanced degree or certificate in a health professions education program.

While there may be some who were born to be great teachers, there are many more who can develop such an ability. And every educator can improve the breadth and depth of his or her understanding of what is known about instructional approaches, the learning sciences, and the evaluation of teachers, learners and programs. In fact, it is critical to do so, because pursuing excellence in teaching is essential to the success of any educational program.

Teachers form a core part of the intellectual capital of a medical school. Outstanding educators not only facilitate the development and assessment of learners, and bring innovative approaches to curriculum design; but they also help the school to attract high caliber students and to enhance the reputation of the school. As everyone knows, teachers create enduring memories that live forever in the minds of the school's alumni.

Importantly, teachers are key communicators of the hidden curriculum, which forms lasting impressions on students and their values, their ethics and their sense of what it means to be a member of a profession. Thus, it is essential that teachers continue to develop, hold themselves to the highest professional and ethical standards, and maintain current knowledge and skill both in their domain of expertise and of new approaches and developments in teaching and mentoring.

So, while it is true that telling someone how to be a better teacher is a most delicate matter, Harden and Laidlaw tackle this task by providing just the right balance of core knowledge and practical advice, evidence and anecdote, art and science. I am confident that you will find this book to be both an engaging read and containing key information and valuable ideas that will enhance and enrich your own teaching.

Steven L. Kanter, MD
Vice Dean, University of Pittsburgh School of Medicine

PREFACE

Over the years there have been requests for a book to be published that complements the courses in medical education which we have run. This is the book. It serves two purposes. It introduces new teachers to the exciting opportunities facing them whether they are working in undergraduate, postgraduate or continuing education. It also assists more experienced teachers to review and assess their own practice and gain a new perspective on how best to facilitate their students' or trainees' learning. We do not claim that the book is comprehensive. More detailed texts on medical education or on education more generally are available and these can be valuable sources of additional information. In writing the book we have taken into consideration the constraints on teachers' time, and the need to produce a book that would be succinct yet useful. Bearing in mind Albert Einstein's view that 'Any intelligent fool can make things bigger and more complex' we have striven to ensure that teachers will not find this book unnecessarily complex.

The information and suggestions offered are based on our extensive experiences in teaching and curriculum planning and in the organisation of faculty development courses in medical education at basic and advanced levels. In other words the content for the book is based on what works in medical education. In writing the book we have had three aims in mind. First, to provide hints drawn from our practical experience that will help teachers to create powerful learning opportunities for their students. In doing so, we have tried to translate what is known from the numerous studies and research in education into readable guidelines for the teacher. Where appropriate we have introduced new techniques that potentially could be adopted for use in a teaching programme. We have tried not to be over-prescriptive, recognising that readers will need to adapt the recommendations to suit their own situation. While retaining a practical focus, our second aim has been to introduce clearly and unambiguously some key basic principles that underpin the practical advice given and that help to inform teaching practice. Effective teaching demands much more than the acquisition of technical skills. An understanding of teaching and learning is essential if the teacher is to be able to respond to a changing situation in the learning context and to the demands over time for change. Recognising that there is no one best method of teaching, our third aim is to assist readers to reflect on and analyse with colleagues the different ways that their work as a teacher or trainer can be approached and their students' or trainees' learning made more effective. What makes teaching exciting is that each situation is different and that through responding to this challenge teachers will achieve more satisfaction and enjoyment in their work.

R. M. Harden
J. M. Laidlaw
Dundee 2012

ABOUT THE AUTHORS

Ronald M. Harden

Professor Ronald Harden graduated from the medical school in Glasgow, UK. He completed training and practised as an endocrinologist before moving full time to medical education. Professor Harden was Professor of Medical Education, Teaching Dean, Director of the Centre for Medical Education and Postgraduate Dean at the University of Dundee. He is currently editor of *Medical Teacher* and General Secretary and Treasurer of the Association for Medical Education in Europe (AMEE).

Professor Harden is committed to developing new approaches to medical education, curriculum planning and teaching and learning. Ideas that he has pioneered include the Objective Structured Clinical Examination (OSCE) which has been universally adopted as a standard approach to assessment of clinical competence. He has published more than 400 papers in leading journals and is co-editor of the best-selling book *A Practical Guide for Medical Teachers*. He has also lectured and run courses on medical education across the globe.

His contributions to excellence in medical education have attracted numerous awards including honorary fellowships of the Royal College of Physicians and Surgeons of Canada and the Royal College of Surgeons in Edinburgh, the Hubbard Award by the National Board of Medical Examiners in the USA, the MILES award by the National University of Singapore, the Karolinska Institutet Prize for Research in Medical Education, the ASME Richard Farrow Gold Medal and the AMEE Lifetime Achievement Award. In addition he was awarded by the Queen the OBE for his services to medical education.

Jennifer M. Laidlaw

Jennifer Laidlaw joined the University of Dundee's Centre for Medical Education in 1975 having previously been a media resource officer for the Royal Bank of Scotland and an innovator of their first distance learning programmes for bank staff.

At the University of Dundee, she initially taught on a Diploma in Medical Education course attended by WHO fellows from the Eastern Mediterranean Region (EMRO). For over 20 years she planned, organised and led courses on medical education both in Dundee and overseas.

She has acted as a medical education consultant for the World Health Organization, the British Council, medical schools and colleges. She has run workshops in Malaysia, the United Arab Emirates, Australia, Egypt, Kuwait, Thailand, Bangladesh, Hungary and Romania.

She provided the educational design for the Centre's distance learning programmes which were distributed to over 50 000 healthcare profession-als, including general practitioners, surgeons, pharmacists, dentists, nurses and physiotherapists. Her postgraduate experience was with junior doctors designing and teaching on induction courses.

She initiated the Twelve Tips series, which continues to be produced by the journal *Medical Teacher*, and provided the educational design for the series Developing the Teaching Instinct produced by the Education Development Unit of the Scottish Council for Postgraduate Medical and Dental Education.

In her teaching, whether it be face-to-face or at a distance, she has applied the FAIR principles that are highlighted in this book. The approach has certainly worked for her.

ACKNOWLEDGEMENTS

The understanding and experiences in medical education which we share in this book have been gained and made immeasurably richer through our association with colleagues such as Willie Dunn, Len Biran, Jack Genn, the late Miriam Friedman Ben-David and the staff of the Centre for Medical Education in Dundee. They have brought to medical education unique perspectives from which we have benefited. We are grateful to all who have shared their experiences and views on medical education with us at conferences we have attended, through papers we have read, and in schools we have visited. Medical education is an applied discipline and only by seeing and experiencing at first hand what works and what does not work have we been able to distil what we believe to be helpful advice.

We are grateful to Dr Steve Kanter who has written the Foreword to this book and the editorial team at Elsevier for their practical help and advice. Jim Glen drew the cartoons which we hope both entertain the reader and help to convey the messages.

INTRODUCTION

'If you have responsibilities for teaching you must develop the skills, attitudes and practices of a competent teacher.'
Good Medical Practice, UK General Medical Council

A CHANGING SCENE

Progress in teaching practice has been relatively modest compared to changes in the practice of medicine that have taken place in the last 100 years, but things are changing. There has been a significant inertia with regard to medical education among medical schools and postgraduate bodies – some for reform and others against change. Issues remain to be tackled such as the continuum of education across the different phases of a doctor's career and the matching of the education programme to the needs of the learner. Other issues have been identified in the Flexner follow-up report by the Carnegie Foundation *Educating Physicians: A Call for Reform of Medical Schools and Residency* (Cooke et al 2010), in the Lancet report *Health professionals for a new century: transforming education to strengthen health systems in an independent world* (Frenk et al 2010) and in *The Future of Medical Education in Canada (FMEC): A Collective Vision for MD Education* report (AFMC 2010).

Medical education and professionalism in teaching, relatively ignored in the past, are on today's agenda for governments, the professions and academics. All recognise the importance of an education programme that equips the doctors of the future with the necessary competencies and keeps doctors in practice up-to-date after qualification. Medical education has to change in order to respond to advances in medicine, alterations in the healthcare delivery system and patient expectations, new learning technologies and developments in educational thinking. There is a move to increase the number and diversity of students taught, and at the same time constrain the costs. All of these are catalysts for change. A time of austerity, as at present, is not a time for modest and incremental change in medical education. More fundamental reform is required. We have seen more integrated and inter-professional curricula with clearly defined learning outcomes and teaching and learning in different contexts such as in the urban and rural communities. The public has different expectations of what they want from the medical practitioner, and there are criticisms of the 'ivory tower' university with demands for medical training to be more authentic and responsive to societal needs. There are pressures for quality assurance, accountability, performance measures and standards in medical education. There are also issues relating to globalisation and, with the increased mobility of doctors, issues relating to international dimensions of medical education. At the same time universities and postgraduate institutions are recognising the business dimensions of their activities. They are competing for students or trainees and may be selling their products globally whether it is a curriculum or set of learning resources or assessment instruments.

THE TEACHER IS IMPORTANT

In responding to the pressures for change, the teacher is critical. It has been argued that teachers are the medical school or postgraduate body's greatest asset. Dan Tosteson, former Dean at Harvard, suggested in 1979 that the most important thing as teachers we have to offer our students is ourselves. There is overwhelming evidence that the quality of the teacher makes a huge difference to the effectiveness and the efficiency of the student's learning. It impacts on this in a number of ways. How a teacher manages small group learning is just as important as the adoption of a small group approach in the curriculum. There is no such thing as bad lectures, only bad lecturers. Almost half a century ago, Sir Derrick Dunlop wrote in 1963 in a publication *The Future of Medical Education in Scotland*, 'It is important to remember that the actual details of the curriculum matter little in comparison to the selection of students and teachers. If these are good any system will work pretty well; if they are indifferent the most perfect curriculum will fail to produce results.' This is equally true today. Teaching is like a clinical skill – if you don't get it right it can have serious implications.

Thomas Good (2010), reviewing research on teaching, illustrated the importance of the teacher, with the analogy of how a chicken dinner with salad, wine and an apple can be a completely different experience as we move from restaurant to restaurant or eat at different homes. While the meal can always be improved by better wine or new ingredients, more important is how the basic ingredients are prepared and presented. As Good outlines, the literature on effective teaching is not based on evidence showing that the most effective teachers bring in new components or better ingredients. Rather the literature indicates that some teachers work with basic ingredients better than others.

If you are a teacher, a trainer, a clinical supervisor, someone with responsibility for a section of a course or a dean, you can make a difference to the quality of your students' or trainees' learning experience. Accrediting bodies such as the General Medical Council in the UK have recognised that all doctors to a greater or lesser extent have teaching responsibilities and have highlighted teaching competence as an important learning outcome in undergraduate and postgraduate programmes. A teacher, to fulfil their educational role, needs to possess or acquire the necessary knowledge, skills and attitudes.

Many medical schools and institutions now recognise good teaching with financial incentives or promotion. Good teaching can bring its own rewards and perhaps the greatest reward is knowing that through teaching the teacher is helping to shape the next generation of doctors. Christa McAuliffe was to be the first teacher in space but died tragically when her spaceship disintegrated 70 seconds after take-off. Earlier, when asked what she did, she replied, 'I touch the future, I teach'.

BEING A GOOD TEACHER

The educational process has three elements: the curriculum, the student and the teacher. Much attention has been paid to the curriculum including the different approaches to teaching, learning and assessment, and to the selection of students and how they can learn more effectively. Less attention has been paid to the teacher. The teacher or trainer is a key element in the creation of the conditions in which learning occurs. (We have used interchangeably throughout the book 'teacher' or 'trainer' and 'student' or 'learner'.) Lawrence Stenhouse, an education guru, suggested that there could be no such thing as curriculum development without teacher development. Good teachers have a range of technical skills, an understanding of basic educational principles, an enthusiasm and passion for teaching and a commitment to evaluating and improving their own teaching. The acquisition of these abilities by a teacher is important.

In teaching, much may be seen as common sense or obvious but experience shows that when it comes to putting it into practice, teachers often flounder and are found wanting. Teachers can learn from experience but this in itself is not enough. It is easy for golfers to go round a golf course practising their mistakes but if the mistakes are never rectified they are unlikely to improve and win the monthly medal! The provision of guidelines for good teaching practice, opportunities for staff development and feedback from students are all key factors that enable teachers to acquire and improve the necessary competencies. There are formal courses on medical education but not everyone can afford the time or the fees to take advantage of them, and a course may not be available that addresses a teacher's specific needs.

HOW THIS BOOK CAN HELP

There is no magic bullet to becoming a competent teacher but this book can point teachers in the right direction. It has been written in the belief that teaching is both a craft and a science and that, with a better understanding of their work, poor teachers can become good teachers and good teachers can become excellent teachers. *Essential Skills for a Medical Teacher: An introduction to teaching and learning in medicine* provides practical advice on four key questions to be addressed by teachers or trainers:

- what should be learned or taught (the learning outcomes)
- how the training or learning programme can be organised (the curriculum)
- how students or trainees can learn most effectively (the teaching and learning methods)
- how the learning can be assessed (assessment).

Four sections of the book are devoted to these key questions, and the responses to them are linked throughout the book. When a new learning approach is introduced, for example, consideration needs to be given to the possible impact on the educational environment, the expected learning outcomes and how students will be assessed. In Section 1 the reader is introduced to some basic educational principles. These provide a valuable lead-in to the sections that follow with the principles revisited in later sections in relation to curriculum planning, teaching and learning methods and assessment. A final section highlights some general conclusions about the teacher's role and anticipates the challenges ahead.

At the start of each section there is an introduction to the chapters and the themes within the section. Each chapter concludes with recommendations for teachers to consider in relation to their own teaching practice. There is also an 'Exploring Further' section where texts are identified that explore a topic in more depth and provide more detailed information and advice. If the reader has a few hours available in a busy schedule then there are suggested readings that can be dipped into. Other readings, including suggested textbooks, require more time.

Teaching is a personal matter. The commitment of teachers and trainers is important if they are to respond adequately to the challenges facing medical education. The work should be enjoyed and not endured. We hope this book will help you, whether you are working with students in the undergraduate curriculum or with trainees in postgraduate or specialist training. Remember, teaching well is more fun than teaching poorly, and everyone is capable of being a good teacher.

REFERENCES

AFMC, 2010. The Future of Medical Education in Canada (FMEC): A Collective Vision for MD Education. The Association of Faculties of Medicine of Canada, Ottawa.

Cooke, M., Irby, D.M., O'Brien, B.C., 2010. Educating Physicians: A Call for Reform of Medical Schools and Residency. Jossey-Bass, San Francisco.

Frenk, J., Chen, L., Bhutta, Z.A., et al., 2010. Health professionals for a new century: transforming education to strengthen health systems in an interdependent world. Lancet 376, 1923–1958.

Good, T.L., 2010. Forty years of research on teaching 1968–2008: What do we know now that we didn't know then? In: Marzano, R.J. (Ed.), On Excellence in Teaching. Solution Tree Press, Bloomington, Indiana, pp. 31–64 (Chapter 2).

Tosteson, D.C., 1979. Learning in Medicine. N. Engl. J. Med. 301, 690–694.

SECTION I
THE ROLES AND COMPETENCIES OF A 'GOOD' TEACHER

'Good teachers are enthusiastic and enjoy teaching. Their enthusiasm for teaching and their subject is infectious.'
Jane Dacre 2003

OVERVIEW

The underlying theme of this book is that the art and skills of teaching can be learned. The good teacher can become an excellent teacher and the poor teacher can become a good teacher.

Chapter 1 What is a good teacher?
Good teachers and trainers are much more than transmitters of information and skills. They facilitate students' learning and they do this in a number of ways. Technical competence and how teachers approach their work are both important.

Chapter 2 Understanding basic educational principles
A teacher is a professional not a technician. An understanding of some basic principles about learning can inform the teacher or trainer in their day-to-day practice.

Chapter 3 Being an enthusiastic and passionate teacher
The good teacher and trainer should have a passion for teaching and the ability to motivate the learner.

Chapter 4 Knowing what works best
Teaching is both a craft and a science. Decisions taken by a teacher or trainer can be informed by evidence as to what works. At the same time, intuition and professional judgement play a key part.

Chapter 5 Checking your performance as a teacher and keeping up-to-date
Teachers should take responsibility for their personal and continuing professional development and regularly assess and review their own competence.

What is a good teacher?

Good teachers and trainers are much more than transmitters of information and skills. They facilitate students' learning and they do this in a number of ways. Technical competence and how teachers approach their work are both important.

WHAT IS EXPECTED OF A TEACHER

Teachers today have a challenging and multifaceted role. Teaching is about much more than the transmission of information to the learner. Teaching encompasses the complex tasks of planning, preparing and delivering a learning programme and assessing whether students have achieved the expected learning outcomes. Students learn all of the time. It is a natural activity. The job of a teacher is to facilitate this by working with the students to:

- clarify the expected learning outcomes
- deliver a programme with appropriate learning opportunities
- support and facilitate the student's learning
- assess the learner's progress in achieving the set goals.

An analogy, in some respects, is the travel agent who, with special knowledge in an area, provides clients with information according to their specific requirements, assists them to explore the range of options that match their needs, arranges the necessary transport and accommodation, and advises on a programme of activities at their destination.

To support the student's learning, the good teacher must have in addition to the necessary subject knowledge, technical skills required for lecturing, facilitating small group discussions, providing feedback, and assessing the student's competence. To do their job effectively and efficiently teachers should have a basic understanding of the educational principles involved. They should also demonstrate the necessary attitudes and professionalism for the job. Here lies a problem. Staff development programmes and texts on the subject frequently address only the technical competencies, or alternatively focus on the educational theory, which may be seen by the practising teacher as of little relevance. The concept of professionalism and attitudes to teaching are largely ignored. It is now recognised that the effective teacher requires a combination of technical competence, an appropriate approach to their teaching, and professionalism in their work as a teacher (Fig. 1.1). These are described in more detail in the chapters that follow.

3

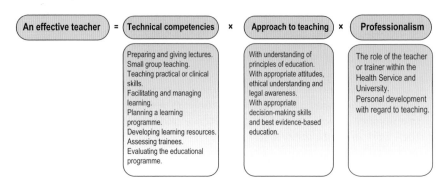

FIG 1.1 The competencies and attributes expected of an effective teacher.

The multiplication symbol has been used in the equation in Figure 1.1 rather than the addition symbol. The implication is that a demonstration of technical competence, no matter how good, on its own is not sufficient. A zero score for the approach to teaching or for professionalism will result in a total score for the rating of the teacher of zero.

Teaching is both an art and a science. Some teachers are instinctively good teachers but others may not be so. The reassuring fact, however, is that the art and science of teaching can be learned. The experienced teacher can develop further their teaching instinct and the new teacher can be helped to acquire this instinct and the necessary competencies, attitudes and professionalism.

What is required of a good teacher will vary to some extent depending on the subject being taught, and in which part of the world the teaching is taking place. There are however certain principles, approaches and views of teaching that are common to the different contexts. We highlight these in this book. It can be argued that the similarities are greater than any differences.

TECHNICAL COMPETENCIES

Eight core areas of technical task-orientated competencies for a teacher are described in Figure 1.1.

A teacher should be competent in:

- preparing and giving lectures or presentations that engage the audience and make use of appropriate technology
- choosing appropriate small group methods and facilitating a small group teaching session
- teaching practical or clinical skills in a variety of settings including the work place
- facilitating and managing the student's learning in a range of settings, giving the learner support to obtain the maximum benefit from the learning opportunities available, helping the student to assess his or her own competence and providing feedback to the learner as necessary

- planning an education programme for the students or trainees that combines appropriate learning opportunities to help them to achieve the expected learning outcomes
- identifying, developing and adapting learning resources for use by students in the form of handouts, study guides or multi-media presentations
- assessing the achievement of learning outcomes by the students or trainees using appropriate technologies including written, performance-based and portfolio assessments
- evaluating the education programme including the use of feedback from the learner and peer assessment.

When teachers are asked in how many of these competencies they would expect a good teacher to excel, the answers varies from all of the competencies to a selected number.

APPROACH TO TEACHING

An effective teacher, in addition to having the necessary technical competencies, approaches their teaching with:

- **An understanding of basic educational principles.** As discussed in Chapter 2, an understanding of basic educational principles helps teachers to adapt the teaching approach to their own situation, to deal with problems and difficulties encountered, and to respond to the need for change as it arises.
- **Appropriate ethics and attitudes.** The ethical standards expected of medical teachers in their work as a teacher or researcher in medical education has been a focus of attention. As discussed in Chapter 3, the teacher's attitude is about much more than ethical behaviour. A key factor in student learning is a teacher's attitude, passion and enthusiasm for the subject and for their teaching.
- **Strategies for decision making.** Paralleling the move to evidence-based medicine, the need for the teacher to make education decisions informed by the best evidence available is very much on today's agenda. At the same time the good teacher has to be able to behave intuitively and to respond appropriately to unexpected situations as they arise in the classroom or work-place learning situation. This is discussed in Chapter 4.

PROFESSIONALISM AND SCHOLARSHIP OF TEACHING

Teachers as professionals should be inquirers into their own competence, should reflect on their own teaching practice, and should audit the quality of their teaching. Teachers have the responsibility to keep themselves up-to-date with current approaches to teaching, and to communicate their own experiences and lessons learned to others. This is discussed in Chapter 5.

Writing in *Scholarship Reconsidered*, Boyer (1990) described teaching as one of the scholarships expected of faculty or staff in a university.

THE ROLES OF THE TEACHER

What is expected of teachers will vary depending on their particular role. Harden and Crosby (2000) have identified twelve roles of a teacher, grouped into six areas (Fig. 1.2):

- information provider in a classroom lecture setting or in a clinical or practical class
- role model on the job in clinical practice or in the teaching context
- learning facilitator or mentor
- assessor of the student's learning and a curriculum evaluator
- curriculum planner or course organiser
- developer of learning resources or producer of study guides.

Roles to the right in Figure 1.2 require more content expertise or knowledge and roles to the left more educational expertise. Roles to the top are associated with face-to-face contact with students and roles to the bottom of the diagram are associated with less student contact. Teaching usually combines several of these roles. It would be unusual to expect a teacher to fulfil all of the roles.

A questionnaire that can be used to assess a teacher's perception of the importance of the twelve roles, their current personal commitment to each role and their preferred personal future commitment is given in Appendix 7.

As will be seen in the chapters that follow, the different roles and responsibilities require of the teacher a range of competencies and attributes. This can be assessed using the grid in Appendix 8.

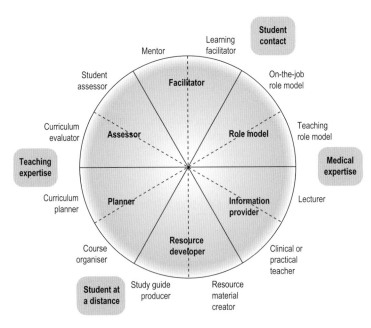

FIG 1.2 The twelve roles of the teacher.

REFLECT AND REACT

1. How effective a teacher are you in terms of, as summarised in Figure 1.1, your technical competencies, your approach to teaching and your professionalism?
2. Think about your own role as a teacher. You may find it of interest to complete the questionnaire in Appendix 7.
3. From your experience as a teacher or learner think about what is expected of a teacher in each of the twelve roles, as summarised in Appendix 8.

EXPLORING FURTHER

IF YOU HAVE A FEW HOURS

Harden, R.M., Crosby, J.R., 2000. AMEE Educational Guide No. 20. The good teacher is more than a lecturer – the twelve roles of the teacher. Med. Teach. 22, 334–347.
A description of the twelve roles of the medical teacher grouped into six areas.

Hatem, C.J., Searle, N.S., Gunderman, R., et al., 2011. The educational attributes and responsibilities of effective medical educators. Acad. Med. 86, 474–480.
This article identifies the skill set of teachers across the medical education curriculum.

Hesketh, E.A., Bagnall, G., Buckley, E.G., et al., 2001. A framework for developing excellence as a clinical educator. Med. Educ. 35, 555–564.
A description of the twelve areas of competence expected of a clinical teacher.

IF YOU HAVE MORE TIME

Boyer, E.L., 1990. Scholarship Reconsidered: Priorities of the Professoriate. John Wiley and Sons, New York.
The classic text that recognised teaching as a scholarly activity.

Skelton, A., 2005. Understanding Teaching Excellence in Higher Education. Routledge, London.
An interesting account of what is expected of an excellent university teacher.

What is a good teacher?

Understanding basic educational principles

A teacher is a professional not a technician. An understanding of some basic principles about learning can inform the teacher or trainer in their day-to-day practice as a teacher or trainer.

BE FAIR TO YOUR STUDENTS

A professional teacher, as we have discussed in the previous chapter, does not operate using a cookbook approach, blindly following a set of rules or procedures. Good teaching, just like any other field of professional endeavour, is best delivered when there is an understanding of the underlying process. Educational researchers have devoted a lifetime to studying education and have described a variety of theories and factors that influence learning. The work in educational psychology described in educational textbooks is often more associated with the experimental laboratory than the reality of practice in the classroom. There are, however, some general principles about learning that can inform what we do as medical teachers.

A comprehensive study of educational theory is out of place in this book and in any case is unlikely to be of interest or relevance to the reader. We have distilled four key principles about effective learning to which teachers can relate in their day-to-day practice. If applied, these principles can improve the effectiveness and efficiency of learning for students or trainees. Most learners in the healthcare professions are capable learners and should have little difficulty in achieving the expected learning outcomes providing they are given some help from their teacher or supervisor.

We have used the acronym FAIR. Be FAIR to your students by providing:

- **Feedback.** Give feedback to students as they progress to mastery of the expected learning outcomes.
- **Activity.** Engage the student in active rather than passive learning.
- **Individualisation.** Relate the learning to the needs of the individual student.
- **Relevance.** Make the learning relevant to the students in terms of their career objectives.

9

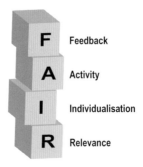

Feedback

Activity

Individualisation

Relevance

FIG 2.1   The FAIR principles for effective learning.

FEEDBACK

Feedback is information communicated to the learner that is intended to modify his or her thinking or behaviour in order to improve learning. Feedback provided by the teacher to the student:

- Clarifies goals. It highlights what is expected of the learner.
- Reinforces good performance. It has a motivating effect on the learner and may reduce anxiety.
- Provides a basis for correcting mistakes. It enables learners to recognise their deficiencies and helps to guide them in their further study.

Knowledge of the extent to which the expected learning outcomes have been achieved will lead the student to more effective and efficient learning. It will provide for learners an insight into their performance that they might not otherwise have. Feedback is part of a two-way communication between a teacher or trainer and the learner. Feedback should be regarded as an essential teaching activity.

It has been demonstrated that academic achievement in classes where effective feedback is provided for students is considerably higher than in classes where this is not so. As Hattie and Timperley (2007) reported, the most powerful single thing that teachers can do to enhance achievement of their students is to provide them with feedback.

Satisfaction studies carried out both with undergraduate students and postgraduate trainees have revealed that one of the commonest complaints students have is that they do not receive meaningful feedback. Too often feedback is omitted or, if provided, is not seen to be helpful.

How to give constructive feedback has been identified by teachers as one of the core competencies thought to be important in their work as a teacher. Much is known about how effective feedback can be provided. It is a skill that can be learned. Here we provide eight evidence-based practical guidelines:

1. *Give an explanation.* In providing feedback, give learners an explanation as to what they did or did not do to meet the expectations. Simply giving a grade or mark in an examination or indicating that learners are right or wrong is less likely to improve their performance. The aim is to help the learner reflect on their performance and to understand the gaps in their learning.

2. *Ensure the feedback is specific.* Provide learners with feedback about their performance against clearly defined learning outcomes. Informing learners how they compare to their peers or informing them in general terms that they lack competence in an area has little value.

3. *Feedback should be non-evaluative.* Feedback should be phrased in as non-evaluative language as possible. It is not helpful, for example, to inform learners that their performance was 'totally inadequate'.

4. *Feedback should be timely and frequent.* Feedback is more effective when learners receive it immediately than when it is delayed and provided in a later class or session. We have found that providing students with a feedback session immediately following an Objective Structured Clinical Examination (OSCE) is a useful and powerful learning experience.

5. *Prepare adequately in advance.* Ensure all the evidence is available with regard to the student's performance before an attempt is made to provide them with feedback. The teacher should be in a position to provide feedback from first-hand experience with the student.

6. *Feedback should help learners to plan their further study.* Assist learners to plan their programme of further learning based on their understanding of where they are at present. This may involve giving them specific reading material or organising further practical or clinical experiences appropriate to their needs.

7. *Help the learner to appreciate the value of feedback and how to interpret it.* A small number of learners may find it difficult to accept and act on feedback provided. One strategy that can help is to ask the learner, before the actual content of the feedback is considered, to reflect orally or in writing on their attitude to being given the feedback.

8. *Encourage learners to provide feedback to themselves.* Feedback is usually thought of as something that is provided exclusively by teachers. Students should be encouraged to assess and monitor their own performance. Ask the learner what they think they have done well and where they think there are problems. Learners can be provided with tools to assist them to assess themselves. Following an OSCE, for example, students can be given a copy of their marked OSCE checklist, a video of their performance and a video demonstrating the expected performance at the OSCE station.

ACTIVITY

A second strategy that has been shown to enhance achievement is active engagement of the learner. Good teachers incorporate active learning into their teaching and learning programme. The principle of active learning is implicit in many of the changes that have taken place in the medical curriculum. These include student-centred approaches, the use of small group work and problem-based learning.

The traditional lecture has been criticised in that the learning is all too often passive with information passed from the lecturer's notes to the student's notes without going through the brain of either.

Evidence demonstrates that where a learner is actively involved in the learning process, the achievements will be significantly enhanced. Learners should be challenged to think and review what they are studying and how new information and skills can be incorporated into their existing knowledge base and skills repertoire. The active learning results in a deeper and more meaningful processing of the learning material with information being stored in the long-term memory. What we need to guard against is 'inert knowledge' – information transmitted to the student that is not used and usually forgotten.

Some learning methods such as simulation and portfolio learning, by their very nature, actively engage the student while others such as the lecture or printed text are frequently associated with passive learning. Almost all learning situations can be transformed from a passive to an active one. Here are some examples:

- Where lectures are scheduled, engage the audience to reflect on and respond to what is being discussed. An electronic audience response system, such as those seen in television game shows, or coloured cards can be used as described in Chapter 21.
- Small group teaching, by its nature, is more interactive but guard against it regressing into mini tutorials. Learners should actively engage with other group members and with the teacher who acts as the facilitator of the discussion rather than the presenter of information – 'the guide on the side rather than the sage on the stage'.
- In the clinical context ensure that learners are not simply passive observers. Learners can be given specific roles and be encouraged to be actively involved in a patient care activity.
- Independent learning resources recommended for use by students, whether in print or online, should be interactive. Available texts or resources can be enriched by the teacher through the addition of meaningful activities that actively engage the student.
- The use of technologies such as models and simulators can contribute to active learning. To assist the learners to make full use of the resources, it is useful to provide support material and guidance in the form of print, audiotapes, video tapes or computer programs. Activities may be programmed into the simulator.
- Ensure that portfolios involve an active reflective process and are not simply a log or rote documentation of activities carried out by the learners. They should not be seen as a chore with no attempt made to distil general principles or practice points. Learners should reflect on the task and document what they have learned in the process.

Whatever the context – whether in the lecture theatre, small group situation, practical laboratory clinical setting or independent learning – scheduled activities should be designed to be meaningful. Clicking to turn a page in an e-learning programme is an activity but it does not contribute to the student's learning. It is important that the teacher and students grasp the purpose or function of an activity and how it contributes to a mastery of the learning outcomes.

The development of student activities can be time consuming but at the same time it is rewarding. The associated cost and resource implications can be justified more easily where the object of the learning is a complex task or a difficult concept, such as gaining an understanding of acid–base balance.

INDIVIDUALISATION

In the present consumer culture, the needs of the individual are being increasingly recognised whether it is in relation to planning a holiday or purchasing a computer. The same should be true of education. We all have different learning needs and learn in different ways.

Teachers have had to cope in medical schools with large classes of students and have had to design the learning experiences and programmes accordingly. As illustrated in Figure 2.2, students, like the raw material entering a factory, pass through a standard process emerging as a product with a uniform specification. There has been little opportunity to cater for the needs of the individual student. Students have different requirements in terms of:

- personal capabilities
- motivation and what drives their learning
- learning goals and career aspirations
- mastery of the course learning outcomes on entry to the course
- learning styles
- the place of learning – on campus or at a distance
- the time of learning.

Students are now less willing to accept teaching and learning opportunities that do not match their needs and help them to achieve their personal learning goals. With the availability of new learning technologies, we need to work towards an 'adaptive learning' programme where the experience offered to students adapts to their personal needs as they work through the programme. Of the four principles mentioned in this chapter, individualisation is probably the most difficult to apply. It is the one where we are likely to see the most change in the next decade.

Today, faced with the challenge of individualising learning, the teacher has a number of options:

- The issue of individualisation can be ignored with the teacher and the education programme addressing the needs of the body of students as a

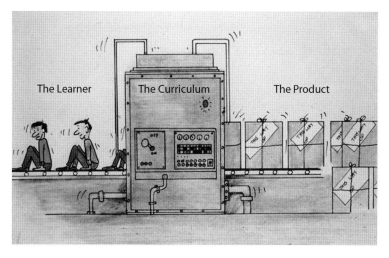

The Learner   The Curriculum   The Product

FIG 2.2   A factory approach with a standard product.

whole. This has disadvantages as illustrated in the following example. An analysis of the examination results in a medical school showed that two thirds of the class answered questions on a specific topic incorrectly. As a response to this finding, a decision was taken to restore a number of lectures on the topic which had previously been omitted from the curriculum. This may or may not address the performance problem with regard to the students who had given the wrong answers to the questions. It penalised however the third of the class who had mastered the subject and for whom the revised lecture course was not appropriate.

- A range of learning opportunities can be provided from which students can select those which best suit their personal needs. The teaching programme may be arranged so that students can choose to attend a lecture on a subject, view a podcast of the lecture, engage in collaborative problem-based learning with their peers, or work independently using an online learning programme. The extent and range of learning opportunities included in the menu for the students will depend on the time and resources available. A move in this direction is supported by the increasing availability of e-learning resources.

- Learning resources or learning opportunities can be adapted or prepared so that the student's learning experience, as they work through the programme, is personalised to their individual needs. If students answer incorrectly a question embedded in a learning programme, or if they indicate they have difficulty understanding the message being conveyed, a further explanation and additional material that addresses the aspect of the topic is provided immediately.

- When learning experiences are scheduled in the programme, such as a session with a simulator, the time allotted for an individual student is not fixed, but is the length of time necessary for the student to master the required skills. Some students or trainees will take longer to master the skills than others.

- With the expansion of medical knowledge and the danger and problem of information overload, students can no longer be provided with in-depth learning in all aspects of medicine. Time can be scheduled in the learning programme when students have a greater element of choice in the subjects studied. Up to a third of the curriculum time may be allocated for electives or student selected components (SSCs). This is discussed further in Chapter 17.

- Portfolio assessment encourages students to create their own learning programme and to demonstrate their learning in relation to the core and other areas they choose to study. This is described in Chapter 31.

RELEVANCE

A major criticism of much of medical education in the past has been a lack of relevance of the subjects taught, particularly in the early years of the medical course. This was highlighted in numerous reports on medical education published throughout the twentieth century. Particular concern was expressed about how the basic sciences were taught with a common criticism that the subjects as taught lacked relevance to the training of a doctor.

Pressures to constantly examine the relevance of what is covered in the curriculum include:

- the rapid expansion of medical knowledge and concerns about information overload
- the introduction of new subjects such as genetics and telemedicine
- important learning outcomes which have been previously ignored such as communication skills and professionalism.

Relevance is an important consideration in curriculum planning, in the preparation of a teaching programme, and in the creation of assessment tools for a number of reasons:

- If students understand why they are addressing a topic they will be more motivated to learn. Adding relevance to teaching creates a powerful and rich experience. In general students learn more rapidly if they are motivated and realise that what they learn will be useful to them in the future.
- More effective learning results when the student is engaged in applying theory to practice. This requires the student to reflect and think about why they are learning a subject, which in turn dramatically improves the effectiveness of their learning. Inert knowledge that is not applied remains only in the short-term memory.
- A set of clinical cases or presentations used as a framework for the curriculum provides a scheme around which students, from the early years of their studies, can construct their learning in the basic and clinical sciences.
- Relevance can be applied as a criterion to inform a decision as to whether a topic or subject should be incorporated in the curriculum. More has to be learned but the time available in the curriculum remains constant.

The engagement of medical students in more authentic learning experiences offers many advantages, but there may be associated difficulties. Teachers in the early years of the curriculum may be equipped to tackle the subjects from the perspective of a basic scientist. They may not have practised as a doctor and may have difficulty in putting the topic into a clinical context.

The curriculum can be designed so that the students' attention is focused on the application of what they are learning to their future practice as a doctor. The following are examples of how relevant and meaningful learning contexts can be created:

- A vertically integrated curriculum with clinical experiences including attachments introduced in the early year of the course (Chapter 15).
- A problem-based approach where students' learning is structured round clinical problems (Chapter 14).
- The use of virtual patients where a student is presented online with a patient whose problem relates to the subject they are studying (Chapter 26).

- A clear statement of expected exit learning outcomes and communication with the student as to how their learning experiences will contribute to their mastery of the learning outcomes (Chapter 19).
- Examinations designed to assess the student in the context of clinical practice. A short patient scenario may be used as the stem for an MCQ in a basic science question paper. Portfolio assessment (Chapter 31) can be designed to support relevance in the student's learning.
- New technologies such as simulators provide for the student a more realistic learning experience (Chapter 25).

REFLECT AND REACT

1. Recognise in your own teaching the importance of feedback. Ask your students or trainees how they perceive the feedback provided by you. By paying attention to feedback, you can promote a culture of positive improvement in your learners.
2. Look at your own teaching and assess the extent to which students are actively engaged in what they perceive as meaningful activities. Documentation in a logbook of the cases they have seen involves the students in an activity, but if the student does not perceive the benefit of the exercise, it can be seen as a waste of time.
3. Individualisation and tailoring a learning programme to meet a student's individual needs offers many benefits but is difficult to achieve in practice. Can you adopt in your own teaching programme any of the suggestions in this chapter that might allow you to take into account the differing needs of your students or trainees?
4. Feedback, activity and individualisation are all key ingredients of a teaching programme, but if relevance is missing your teaching is unlikely to be successful. Do you pay sufficient attention to ensuring that students recognise the relevance of their learning experiences?

EXPLORING FURTHER

IF YOU HAVE A FEW HOURS

Harden, R.M., Laidlaw, J.M., 1992. Effective Continuing Education: The CRISIS Criteria. AMEE Guide No. 4. Med. Educ. 26, 408–422.
The CRISIS Criteria – Convenience, Relevance, Individualisation, Self-Assessment, Interest and Systematic – address similar educational principles to those described in the FAIR criteria. Examples are given of each of the principles in continuing education.

Hattie, J., Timperley, H., 2007. The power of feedback. Review of Educational Research 77, 81–112.
An important review of the educational uses of feedback.

Kaufman, D.M., 2010. Applying educational theory in practice. In: Cantillon, P., Wood, D. (Eds.), ABC of Learning and Teaching in Medicine. second ed. Wiley-Blackwell, Oxford (Chapter 1).
A short and helpful description of how to bridge the gap between education theory and practice.

Laidlaw, J.M., Harden, R.M., 1987. Impact of technology on the education of health care professionals. Int. J. Technol. Assess. Health Care 3, 67–82.
A description of the FAIR principles.

IF YOU HAVE MORE TIME

Biggs, J., Tang, C., 2007. Teaching for Quality Learning at University, third ed. Open University Press, Maidenhead. *This text illustrates how theory applied with a delicate touch enables teachers to transform their practice.*

Rogers, A., 2002. Teaching Adults, third ed. Open University Press, Maidenhead. *A classic text, which covers basic principles as well as providing useful hints for teachers.*

2

Understanding basic educational principles

Being an enthusiastic and passionate teacher

The good teacher and trainer should have a passion for teaching and the ability to motivate the learner.

WHAT IS A PASSIONATE TEACHER?

The reader of this book will appreciate how important it is for a teacher to have the technical skills necessary to teach students effectively and efficiently – skills such as delivering a lecture, managing small group learning, or preparing an assessment exercise. We will deal with the different skills later in the book, but having only the technical skills is not enough. Good teachers need to demonstrate a passion for their teaching if they are to motivate their students to learn. The passionate teacher conveys an enthusiasm for the subject and for their teaching. Student surveys have found that the 'master lecturer' not only presents the subject matter with clarity, but also conveys the content with enthusiasm and excitement. 'All effective teachers' suggests Day, 'have a passion for the subject, a passion for their pupils, and a passionate belief that who they are and how they teach can make a difference to their pupils' lives, both in the moment of teaching and in the days, weeks, months and even years afterwards' (Day and Hadfield 2004). The late George Miller described the worst teachers not as those who knew less or taught less but rather as those who were uninterested in their students.

In his book *The Passionate Teacher*, Fried (2001) argues 'Only when teachers bring their passions about teaching and life into their daily work can they dispel the fog of passive compliance or active disinterest that surrounds so many students'. He goes on to distinguish passionate teaching from mere idiosyncrasies or foibles. These may make the teacher memorable for their students, but this is different from the passion we are describing. As Whitehead argued in his classic 1929 text *The Aims of Education*, 'The University imparts information, but it imparts it imaginatively… A university which fails in this respect has no reason for existence. This atmosphere for excitement arising from imaginative consideration transforms knowledge. A fact is no longer a bare fact: it is invested with all its possibilities. It is no longer a burden on the memory: it is energizing as a poet of our dreams and as the architect of our purposes. Imagination is not to be divorced from the facts: it is a way of illuminating the facts'.

DOES IT MATTER?

Does passion matter in teaching? The short answer is 'yes'. Effective teaching is the result of a combination of many factors but passion is at the heart of what good teaching is about. Teachers' passion and enthusiasm for their students' learning is important. Passion and enthusiasm are highlighted in studies of the skills and attributes of excellent teachers. The word 'passion' features regularly in students' descriptions of their best teachers – both the passion teachers have for their subject and the passion they have for sharing their learning with their students. In one study of medical students' perceptions as to what makes an effective medical teacher, the two highest-ranking attributes selected by both senior and junior students were 'is passionate about teaching' and 'motivates and inspires the students' (Kua et al 2006). A review of exemplary university teachers found that they enjoyed teaching, showed enthusiasm for their subject, and made an earnest attempt to promote students' learning (Hativa et al 2001). Passion in teaching is not a luxury or a frill that we can do without – it is the key element in students' learning. When the quality of students' learning is compared in different situations, the differentiating factor is frequently found to be the passion of the teacher – more than their knowledge of subject matter, more than the teaching strategy adopted, and more than the learning technology incorporated.

EVERYONE CAN BE A PASSIONATE TEACHER

Passionate teaching does not require exceptional ability although it is not found in teachers as commonly as one might hope. Fried argues that it is not just a personality trait that some people have and others have not: it is something that can be discovered and learned. You may not be able to be taught how to be a passionate teacher but you can learn how to be one.

Bringing passion to teaching is not easy – it is challenging but it can be done. Depending on your personality your passion can emerge in different ways. Teachers do not have to be extroverted or flamboyant in their presentations to be thought of as passionate about content. They can be reserved and refined in their delivery and still convince the learner of their enthusiasm and commitment to the subject and to the learning.

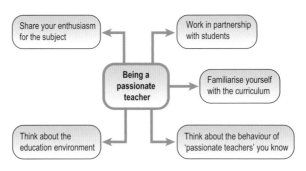

FIG 3.1   How to be a passionate teacher.

Here are suggestions, some taken from the work of Fried, that may help:

- Think about how in your teaching you can share your enthusiasm for your subject with your students.
- Let your students see that you are working in partnership with them to support their learning and not just as an expert standing aloof.
- Think back to the teachers who you most respected and learned from when you were a student. What was it about their teaching that inspired you?
- Think about the aspect of your work as a teacher that gives you the greatest satisfaction. Could you develop this further?
- Don't be surprised if you come across cynics who will try to damp your enthusiasm. Expect to hear comments like 'You've only got a short time to teach on the subject so don't get carried away' or 'Your ideas will never work as there are too many students in the class' or 'We don't have enough resources for you to do that'. Keep in mind that most obstacles put in your way are surmountable.
- Create an appropriate learning environment that manifests interpersonal warmth, empathy, support for students' self esteem, patience and a sense of humour.
- Care for and have a keen interest in the development of your students and feel responsible for their success and for their intellectual and moral well-being.
- Have a deep commitment to provide the best opportunities for each student based on their individual needs. Think about the potential of each student for whom you are responsible and how you might build on their individual strengths.
- It helps to be enthusiastic about your teaching if you are familiar with the curriculum, how your own teaching fits in, and why some topics are given more weight than others. (This can guard against your passion for teaching being stifled or frustrated when you find that the time allocated for your subject has been reduced.)
- Serving on a curriculum committee or course planning team gives you an added insight that you will find helpful.
- If you teach in the context of an integrated or problem-based curriculum, you may find that you have less control over what is taught, and may have to conform to the set teaching strategies. Understand that these approaches have potential advantages and can play an important part in the students' learning.

STRESS AND BURN OUT

With competing pressures for time and demands from the students and the curriculum, teaching can be stressful. Even the most enthusiastic teacher may be stressed and over time can be subject to 'burn out'. This is associated with increased feelings of emotional exhaustion and fatigue, the development of negative cynical attitudes towards students, and the tendency for teachers to evaluate themselves negatively resulting in a feeling of lack of personal accomplishment. Teachers may at times feel overwhelmed with the challenges and workload facing them. A better understanding of their work as a teacher and how the different tasks faced can be tackled may help the teacher to seek assistance if it remains a problem.

REFLECT AND REACT

1. Recognise that much can be achieved by teachers who love to teach and by students who want to learn.
2. Remember that there is no place for teaching by humiliating and patronising students, but there is a place for teachers who demonstrate a passion for their teaching.
3. Are you considered by your students and colleagues to be a passionate teacher, filling them with enthusiasm for your subject? Consider whether with benefit you could adopt some of the strategies outlined above.
4. Are you fully committed to the performance of each student and to the extent to which they are achieving their individual potential? Do students perceive you as someone who is there to help and support them?

EXPLORING FURTHER

IF YOU HAVE A FEW HOURS

Hativa, N., Barak, R., Simhi, E., 2001. Exemplary university teachers. Knowledge and beliefs regarding effective teaching dimensions and strategies. The Journal of Higher Education 72, 699–729.
A review of the attributes of effective teachers.

Kua, E.H., Voon, F., Hoon, C., et al., 2006. What makes an effective medical teacher? Perceptions of medical students. Med. Teach. 28, 738–741.
A short description of the evaluation by students of what makes an effective teacher in medicine.

IF YOU HAVE MORE TIME

Day, C., Hadfield, M., 2004. A Passion for Teaching. Routledge, London.
A description of the importance of being a passionate teacher, and what is required.

Fried, R.L., 2001. The Passionate Teacher: A Practical Guide. Beacon Press, Boston.
A description of a passionate teacher in the context of primary and secondary education that still has meaning in the education of medical students.

Whitehead, A.N., 1929. The Aims of Education and Other Essays. The Free Press, New York.
A classic text still worth dipping into.

Knowing what works best

Teaching is both a craft and a science. Decisions taken by a teacher or trainer can be informed by evidence as to what works. At the same time, intuition and professional judgement play a key part.

EVIDENCE–INFORMED TEACHING

An effective teacher, as highlighted in the previous chapter, requires a set of technical competencies, a basic understanding of educational principles and a passion for teaching, but that is not the end of the matter. There is something else to consider. There is a need for the teacher to openly accept that there may be different and possibly more effective methods of teaching than those they are currently employing. They should not assume that the methods by which they have been taught or those they are currently using are the best.

Doctors are encouraged, as far as possible, to make decisions about the diagnosis and management of their patients on the basis of the evidence of what works and what does not work. This is the key principle of the evidence-based medicine (EBM) movement in health care. Evidence-based education – or probably more appropriate, evidence-informed education – has a similar objective. Teachers should make conscientious explicit and judicious use of evidence as to what works and does not work in their teaching practice. This involves teachers integrating their individual expertise as a teacher with the best available external evidence. Teachers need to question whether a new approach advocated will prove better or worse than the traditional approach which it would be replacing. The concept of evidence-based decision-making was one of the three fundamental principles incorporated in the Carnegie 'Teachers for a New Era' initiative in the USA.

A 'PHOG' APPROACH

Decisions in medical education in the past have been made on what might be called a 'PHOG' approach, with decisions based on the *prejudices* of the teacher, *hunches* of what works best, personal *opinion* and *guesses* as to the most suitable approach.

Sixteen years ago, Cees van der Vleuten at Maastricht highlighted a paradox in medical education. 'I noticed that my new colleagues – clinical and biomedical researchers – had the same academic values as I did, which reassured me

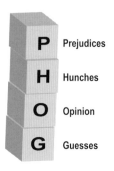

FIG 4.1 The PHOG approach to teaching decisions.

and made me feel comfortable. However I quickly noticed something peculiar; the academic attitudes of the researchers seemed to change when educational issues were discussed. Critical appraisal and scientific scrutiny were suddenly replaced by personal experiences and beliefs and sometimes by traditional values and dogmas.'

Today the need for evidence-informed teaching has been widely accepted, even if it has not been fully implemented in practice. A recent curriculum document from Maastricht, for example, describes the new Maastricht curriculum as an 'evidence-based curriculum'.

WHAT IS EVIDENCE?

What counts as evidence is a difficult question. Relevant evidence may come from professional experience and professional judgement as well as from formal experimental or quasi-experimental research studies. Evidence to inform your decisions as a teacher can come from a variety of sources:

- **Your own personal experience.** As a professional you should inquire into what works for you in your own setting and how the teaching and learning process could be improved.
- **The experience and examples of colleagues.** A key factor in the introduction of the OSCE into medical schools in South Africa was the participation and experiences by teachers as external examiners in an OSCE in another school.
- **Experiences reported in the literature or presented at educational meetings.** Paul Worley described how eight students at Flinders Medical School in Australia received their clinical training in a rural community rather than in a teaching hospital and how they performed in the end of course assessment as well as or better than their colleagues. Despite the relatively small number of students studied, this provided useful evidence and encouragement for teachers interested in developing community-based teaching in their own school.
- **A published review, guide or editorial on a topic.** The Association for Medical Education in Europe (AMEE) guide on Faculty Development

by Michelle McLean and co-workers (2008), for example, provides a helpful summary of experiences with faculty development and how faculty development programmes are best delivered.
- **A systematic review.** Systematic reviews, such as those published by the Best Evidence Medical Education (BEME) collaboration (www. BEMEcollaboration.org), use a systematic and transparent methodology and draw on the collective findings from primary research in specific topics to better inform education practice. The BEME systematic review on simulation, for example, identified ten features that improve learning when high fidelity simulators are used.

SEARCHING FOR EVIDENCE

Searching for evidence to inform best practice in medical education is a complex undertaking. BEME guide No. 3 by Alex Haig and Marshall Dozier (2003) provides a comprehensive overview of relevant information sources. This includes core bibliographic databases such as Medline, Embase, CINHAL (Cumulative Index to Nursing and Allied Health Literature), ERIC (The Education Resource Information Centre), BEI (The British Education Index) and PsycINFO; other less well known databases; and the grey literature which includes print and electronic reports not commercially produced and newsletters, theses and committee reports. The guide describes how to undertake a search and illustrates the process with a number of examples.

EVALUATING EVIDENCE

The QUESTS criteria for the assessment of evidence have been described (Harden et al 1999). These may be of help when you think about the value of evidence you identify:

- **The Quality of the evidence.** This relates to the type of evidence or research method and the rigour of the study. Qualitative methods have a place alongside quantitative approaches. The randomised controlled trial may in practice not yield the best evidence.
- **The Utility of the evidence.** The utility is the extent to which the approach described in the research studies will need to be adapted for use in your own practice. Research on problem-based learning (PBL) for example may be based on a small group size of eight students who meet formally as a group three times per week. The results and conclusions may have to be interpreted with caution if your group size is significantly larger and the meetings less frequent.
- **The Extent of the evidence.** The number of studies reported and the size or extent of the individual studies are relevant. Evidence from a single case study that a new approach has worked well is helpful but it is useful to have this confirmed.
- **The Strength of the evidence.** It is important to distinguish between statistical significance and practical significance.

- **The Target.** This relates to whether what has been assessed as the outcome in a research study matches your own expected outcomes. The evidence may be less relevant because the study addresses a different question from the one in which you are interested. You might be interested for example in the costs and logistics of implementing a new assessment procedure while the reported research has, as its aim, an evaluation of the effect of the assessment on the students' learning.
- **The Setting or context for the study.** Geographical considerations or the phase of the curriculum may be important factors when interpreting any results. There is no such thing as context-free evidence and research findings need to be interpreted in relation to the context in which the research studies were conducted.

The value of reported evidence and the conclusions drawn from it can be considered as the sum of the power of the evidence (the quality, the extent and the strength) and the relevance of the evidence to your teaching practice (the utility, the target and the setting).

BEST EVIDENCE MEDICAL EDUCATION

Evidence-informed teaching is a philosophy that has two elements. First, it involves teachers not taking for granted that their current practice is optimal. Second, evidence should be sought that will inform decisions as to the most effective teaching approach. There is a widely held view amongst clinicians, medical researchers and medical teachers that evidence to inform decisions relating to teaching is not available. This is not the case. Often those who are concerned about the lack of evidence have either not looked for it or have looked in the wrong places! For the most part, the recommendations in this book as they relate to educational strategies such as feedback, to teaching tools such as simulators, and to assessment methods such as the OSCE, are informed by evidence.

The BEME collaboration was established with the aim of helping teachers make decisions about their teaching practice on the best evidence available. Systematic reviews have been produced on a wide range of topics and these provide information about what works, in what circumstances, and for whom. The reviews can help teachers to base their practice on available evidence.

The level of evidence available to inform decisions about day-to-day practice will vary. We are certainly not at the extreme right end of the evidence continuum shown in Figure 4.2, nor are we at the left end. As we learn more and more about what we do as teachers there will be a move towards the right.

INTUITION AND TEACHING

We return to our earlier assertions that medical education is both a science and an art. While an evidence-based approach to teaching is of value, intuition by teachers in their professional practice also has an important, although less well recognised, part to play. Teaching involves the performance of complex

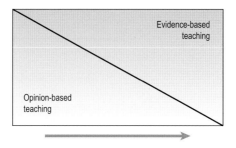

FIG 4.2 The evidence continuum in teaching.

and diverse skills in real time and in contexts that are sometimes unpredictable and constantly evolving. Experienced teachers often cannot explain what they do and why they are doing it. This is not surprising as much of what a teacher does is intuitive – a reaction at the time to students' responses. Intuition can be thought of as the tacit knowledge built by the teacher out of accumulated information and experience. All teachers will need at times to use intuition when making decisions about their teaching practice.

CONCLUSION

Teaching is not simply the adoption of a 'cook book of recipes' developed by others. Teaching and professional judgement needs to be combined with the understanding of the best evidence available so that the teacher can arrive at the correct decision and take the appropriate action.

REFLECT AND REACT

1. With regard to your teaching, consider where you are on the continuum between opinion-based and evidence-based approaches, as shown in Figure 4.2, and whether you might move further to the right.
2. Look at a BEME review, for example BEME review No. 4 on Simulation, and assess whether the conclusions have any relevance to your own teaching.
3. The next time you read an article, assess the implications of the evidence for your own practice in terms of the QUESTS criteria.

EXPLORING FURTHER

IF YOU HAVE A FEW HOURS

Haig, A., Dozier, M., 2003. Systematic Searching for Evidence in Medical Education. BEME Guide No. 3. AMEE, Dundee.
A valuable guide to searching the literature for evidence in medical education.

Harden, R.M., Grant, J., Buckley, G., Hart, I.R., 1999. Best Evidence Medical Education. BEME Guide No. 1. AMEE, Dundee.

A summary of the best-evidence medical education concept and the factors influencing the need to move to evidence-based teaching.

Issenberg, S.B., McGaghie, W.C., Petrusa, E.R., 2004. Features and Uses of High-fidelity Medical Simulations That Lead to Effective Learning. BEME Guide No. 4. AMEE, Dundee.
An example of a BEME systematic review.

IF YOU HAVE MORE TIME

Atkinson, T., Claxton, G., 2000. Intuitive Practitioner: On the Value of Not Always Knowing What One is Doing. Open University Press, Maidenhead.
An account of the importance of intuition in a teacher.

McLean, M., Cilliers, F., Van Wyk, J.M., 2008. Faculty development: yesterday, today and tomorrow. AMEE Guide No. 33. Med. Teach 30, 555–584.
Frameworks for designing, implementing and evaluating faculty development programmes.

www.BEMEcollaboration.org.
The BEME website is a useful collection of information about BEME. It also contains reviews and information about evidence-based teaching.

Checking your performance as a teacher and keeping up-to-date

5

Teachers should take responsibility for their personal continuing professional development and regularly assess and review their own competence.

Teaching is a professional activity that requires:

- mastery of the subject matter that is being taught
- mastery of approaches to teaching that result in students' effective and efficient learning.

It should be apparent from the earlier chapters that teaching is an immensely complex and multifaceted activity that involves a wide range of competencies and attributes. Teachers, if they are to meet their responsibilities, require a range of technical skills that equip them to impart knowledge, teach practical skills, assess students, conduct small group sessions and facilitate students' learning in a range of contexts. These technical skills represented by the inner circle in Figure 5.1 are covered more fully in later chapters of the book. The teacher is a professional and not simply a technician. As described in the earlier chapters in this section, teachers have to approach their work with an understanding of the underpinning educational principles, with the necessary passion and appropriate attitudes, and using a combination of evidence-based decision-making and intuition (the middle circle in Figure 5.1).

In this chapter we focus on the personal development and professionalism of a teacher. This is the outer circle in Figure 5.1. Key professional responsibilities include the need for teachers to:

- reflect upon and be aware of their own strengths and weaknesses as a teacher and to be an inquirer into their own competence
- keep up-to-date with new approaches to teaching and learning
- recognise that the teacher is part of a team which involves collaborating with others engaged in the education process.

A general statement of the values and commitments of a teacher that embody the principles of professionalism is given in Appendix 1.

ENQUIRING INTO YOUR OWN COMPETENCE

As a professional, a key task for teachers is to take responsibility for the quality of their teaching and for the assessment of their own competence as a teacher. In choosing to read this book readers have demonstrated an interest

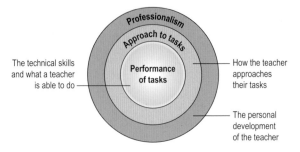

FIG 5.1 Three-circle model of the competencies required of a teacher.

in teaching and hopefully in their own performance as a teacher. In some areas it should be apparent whether a teacher has the required competencies. The expertise necessary to set appropriate standards for assessment procedures or to prepare an e-learning programme are obvious. In other areas, such as lecturing or the facilitation of learning in small groups, the level of expertise required may be less clear.

Most teachers at some stage in their career will have given one or more lectures, run a small group discussion or counselled a student or trainee, without necessarily having reflected on their performance in relation to the task. Self-assessment with an assessment of personal strengths and weaknesses is notoriously difficult. There is good evidence that the poorer performer is more likely to make an over-inflated assessment of their competence. The teacher may believe that he or she has given an outstanding lecture while in practice students find the lecture incomprehensible, boring and irrelevant. A teacher may use a small group session to express his or her own views and thoughts on a topic without appreciating that he or she has failed to engage the students actively in discussion and to stimulate their reflection. The teacher may think that his or her counselling session and feedback provided for the student or trainee in difficulty has gone well, while the opposite is the case and the student is left without any real understanding of his or her problems and what can be done to remedy them. Here are some suggestions that may help teachers to assess their teaching prowess:

- **Stop and reflect on your own performance as a teacher.** By reading this book you have started this process.
- **Study feedback from students** about your performance. Students' views are obtained commonly through a questionnaire or a focused discussion. Feedback should address your coverage of the topic and your method of delivery and presentation skills. The information obtained can be useful, but it has to be treated with an element of caution. In the classic example of what has been termed the 'Dr Fox Effect', a professional actor, unbeknown to the students, was briefed to give an entertaining lecture that was educationally poor. It was subsequently rated highly by students!
- **Obtain feedback from colleagues.** Peer evaluation of teaching is now standard practice in many medical schools. It is important that the feedback provided is constructive rather than destructive. Such feedback is easier to obtain if you are working as part of a team. If you know your peers well, you may be less inhibited to ask for their comments and more likely to receive and accept useful feedback on your performance.

- **Record or videotape your teaching.** This may be useful, and idiosyncrasies and defects in your teaching may become obvious to you. You can assess your performance on your own or with a colleague.
- **Assess whether your students have achieved the expected learning outcomes.** One measure is how well your students perform in written or clinical examination questions relating to the part of the training programme for which you are responsible. This information may not be readily available to you.
- **Assess whether you have influenced your student's or trainee's career choice and subsequent career.** This is also a difficult result to measure.
- **Study measurements of the educational environment** in your institution. Reflect on the possible impact of your teaching on the results.
- **Participate in conferences on medical education.** Participation in educational activities provides you with the opportunity to compare your teaching practice with that of colleagues. This can help you identify aspects of your own teaching performance which you might wish to improve upon.

KEEPING UP-TO-DATE

Medical education, just like medicine and healthcare delivery, is constantly changing. Over the past decade significant developments have taken place with curriculum planning including moves to outcome-based education and inter-professional education; with assessment including the wider use of port-folio assessment and standard setting; and with new learning technologies including high fidelity simulators, virtual patients and the use of the internet.

Teachers in medicine must keep up-to-date in their subject area and, in addition, keep abreast of developments and new approaches to education that may be relevant to their teaching practice. There are different ways of keeping up-to-date and we have listed some of them. Teachers should choose the approach that works best for them.

- **Textbooks.** A growing number of books are available that cover, in more depth than is possible in this book, topics such as curriculum planning, teaching and learning methods, and assessment. A companion volume that discusses some aspects in more detail is *A Practical Guide for Medical Teachers*.
- **Journals.** Most teachers keep abreast of the journals relating to their own specialty, but it is unlikely that the discipline-based journals provide adequate coverage of medical education. Key international journals in the field of medical education are *Medical Teacher*, *Medical Education*, *Teaching and Learning in Medicine* and *Academic Medicine*. You may find more specialised education journals in your own area of teaching such as *Education for Primary Care*, *Anatomical Sciences Education* or *Medical Science Education*.
- **Newsletters.** Many professional organisations produce newsletters that help to keep their members up-to-date with education developments.
- **Guides and reports.** The Association for Medical Education in Europe (AMEE) publishes a series of guides designed to keep the practising

teacher informed about contemporary medical education practice (www.amee.org). Systematic reviews of evidence relating to topics in medical education are published by the Best Evidence Medical Education (BEME) collaboration (www.bemecollaboration.org).

- **Online information.** Information on a range of education topics can be accessed using a search engine such as Google, by joining a list-serv such as DrEd.com, through an online education community such as MedEdWorld (www.MedEdWorld.org) or by following an education blog.
- **Conferences and meetings.** Attendance at a local, national or international conference or meeting where the theme is medical education is a popular way of keeping up to date. Some meetings such as the annual meeting of AMEE include in their programme workshops and master class sessions on a range of medical education topics.
- **Courses on medical education.** An increasing number of courses on medical education are available delivered face to face or at a distance. These may be of short duration or more extended and lead to an award of a certificate, diploma or master's degree in medical education.
- **Membership of professional education associations or communities of practice.** One way of keeping up-to-date is to join a professional organisation committed to medical education. This may be a regional educational organisation such as the Association for the Study of Medical Education (ASME) in the UK, the Spanish Society for Medical Education (SEDEM) in Spain, the Netherlands Association for Medical Education (NVMO) in the Netherlands, or the Canadian Association for Medical Education (CAME) in Canada or an international organisation such as AMEE or the International Association of Medical Science Educators (IAMSE). Membership may include a subscription to a medical education journal, registration for conferences, and access to other membership services. It is worthwhile considering joining a network of medical educators such as MedEdWorld.org, which is an online global network of teachers in the healthcare professions who are committed to sharing ideas, resources and expertise in the field of medical education.

As teachers we have a responsibility through one or more of these approaches to keep up-to-date with what we are expected to teach, how our students can best learn, how the achievement of the learning outcomes can be assessed and how the educational activities can be best organised into a meaningful programme or curriculum.

WORKING AS A MEMBER OF A TEAM

With the increased sophistication and specialisation in medical education it is likely that, whatever activity teachers are engaged in, they will need to collaborate with others whose content or education expertise complements their own. If you are working in assessment, it is likely that you will need to collaborate with someone who has the necessary psychometric or standard setting expertise. If you are developing an e-learning programme, you will need to work with an instructional designer and a computer technologist.

An evaluation some years ago of a UK government Teaching and Learning Technology initiative found that only projects that had content, education and technology experts collaborating together were successful.

The moves towards more vertical and horizontal integration in the curriculum, to outcome-based education and to problem-based learning necessitate basic scientist and clinician teachers working more closely together. The greater emphasis on inter-professional education and work-based learning requires collaboration between teachers and practitioners in the different professions.

An atmosphere of collegiality amongst teachers is important and has been shown to contribute to student achievement. Teachers need to be supportive of and courteous and respectful to each other and demonstrate that they work together as a member of a team.

REFLECT AND REACT

1. Reflect on how you obtain information with regard to your effectiveness as a teacher. Consider the different sources of information listed in this chapter. What are your strengths and weaknesses?
2. Think about how you keep up-to-date in your own discipline or field of interest. Can similar methods be adopted with regard to your responsibilities as a teacher?
3. As a teacher do you work as a member of a team? Do you meet informally with your peers? Are you a member of a curriculum or programme committee? You might consider whether further collaboration with colleagues could be beneficial.
4. Think about your professionalism as a teacher. Could you sign up to the Teacher's Charter in Appendix 1?

EXPLORING FURTHER

IF YOU HAVE A FEW HOURS

McGaghie, W.C., 2010. Scholarship, Publication and Career Advancement in Health Professions Education. AMEE Educational Guide No. 43. AMEE, Dundee. *A description of what scholarship as a teacher in medicine means.*

McLean, M., Cilliers, F., van Wyk, J.M., 2010. Faculty Development: Yesterday, Today and Tomorrow. AMEE Educational Guide No. 33. AMEE, Dundee.

A guide that will help those who have the task of preparing faculty for their roles in teaching and education.

IF YOU HAVE MORE TIME

Carr, D., 2005. Professionalism and Ethics in Teaching (Professional Ethics). Routledge, London.

A discussion of professionalism as it relates more generally to teaching.

SECTION 2
LEARNING OUTCOMES AND OUTCOME-BASED EDUCATION

'No man can be a good teacher unless he has feelings of warm affection toward his pupils and a genuine desire to impart to them what he himself believes to be of value.'
Bertrand Russell

OVERVIEW

The first task for a teacher is to consider the expected learning outcomes for the programme or course where they have a teaching responsibility.

Chapter 6 The need for an outcome-based approach
An important trend is the move from an emphasis on the process of teaching and learning to the product and what is achieved.

Chapter 7 Specifying learning outcomes and competencies
A range of approaches can be used to identify and define the expected learning outcomes.

Chapter 8 Describing and communicating the learning outcomes
Different frameworks or models can be used to categorise and communicate learning outcomes.

Chapter 9 Implementing an outcome-based approach in practice
Outcome-based education requires two things. The learning outcomes need to be identified and specified. Decisions about the curriculum must be based on the specified outcomes.

The need for an outcome-based approach

An important trend is the move from an emphasis on the process of teaching and learning to the product and what is achieved.

WHAT IS OUTCOME-BASED EDUCATION (OBE)?

The most important responsibility teachers have is to identify the learning outcomes or competencies expected of their students or trainees and to ensure that these can be achieved in the education programme.

Traditionally medical education has focused on teaching methods such as the lecture and small group work, on the design of the curriculum and whether, for example, it was community-based or integrated, and on the assessment of the learner and the different approaches adopted. What has been described as the most important trend in medical education in the past decade is the move towards an outcome-based approach where the emphasis is on the product of the learning rather than on the process. Outcome-based education (OBE) is a performance-based approach at the cutting edge of curriculum development and offers a powerful way of changing and managing medical education.

OBE requires:

- The learning outcomes expected at the end of training and at the end of each phase of training to be clearly stated, explicit and communicated to all concerned including teachers, students and other stakeholders such as employers in the health service.
- Decisions about the curriculum, including the content, the educational strategies, the teaching methods and the assessment, to be based on the agreed learning outcomes. The learning outcomes define the process of what is taught, how it is taught and how it is assessed (Fig. 6.1).
- A collectively endorsed vision that reflects a commitment that students will succeed and that their achievement of the exit outcomes will be demonstrated before they leave the programme of training.

The concept of OBE was promoted by Spady (1994). He defined OBE as 'a way of designing, developing, delivering and documenting instruction in terms of its intended goals and outcomes'. Spady suggested that 'Exit outcomes are a critical factor in designing the curriculum. You develop the curriculum from the outcomes you want students to demonstrate, rather

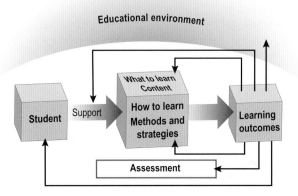

FIG 6.1 Curriculum decisions are based on the learning outcomes.

than writing objectives for the curriculum you already have'. OBE can be summed up as 'results-orientated thinking'. This shift towards OBE is at least in part analogous to the total quality movement in business and manufacturing.

WHY OBE HAS BEEN ADOPTED

OBE offers major advantages, some of which are obvious:

- **OBE highlights the competencies to be achieved.** What matters are the competencies and abilities achieved by doctors, including their knowledge, skills and attitudes, rather than how they were trained or how they acquired these competencies. This has been described as 'education for capability'. In the analogy of buying a car, the customer is more interested in how the car performs, in its features and petrol consumption and in how easily it can be maintained rather than in the details of the car manufacturing process. As Thomas Fuller noted 'A good archer is not known by his arrows but by his aim'.
- **OBE is necessary given the rapid advances in medicine.** Knowledge in the biomedical field is doubling every 18 months. It is no longer feasible, given this information explosion, to cover in the curriculum all aspects of a subject. While the amount of knowledge has greatly increased, the length of the undergraduate curriculum has remained the same at 4, 5 or 6 years' duration. It is now more important than ever that we agree as teachers and advise our students about the core competencies and knowledge we expect them to master.
- **OBE ensures consideration is given to important topics that otherwise might be neglected.** Potentially important topics in the curriculum such as attitudes and professionalism, communication skills, health promotion, team working, patient safety and management of errors have in the past been neglected. OBE helps to ensure that careful consideration is given to these and other key topics.

- **OBE emphasises accountability and transparency in medical education.** To meet demands for greater accountability, quality assurance and transparency are features of medical education today. A clear statement of the learning outcomes achieved is required. An OBE approach to curriculum planning encourages a debate as to the purpose of medical education and what is required of a 'good doctor'. This may include, in addition to the provision of quality care for individual patients, an element of social responsibility or accountability in medicine and the development of the doctor as a global citizen (Hodges 2009).
- **OBE points students in the right direction.** OBE provides a robust framework for the curriculum and can be thought of as the glue that holds the curriculum together. It is consistent with a move to a student-centred approach and provides students with a clearer idea of what is expected of them. Traditionally, when students embarked on their medical training it was more like a 'magical mystery tour'. They lacked an understanding of what was expected of them at the different stages of their education. The provision of a clear set of learning outcomes empowers the students and engages them more actively with the curriculum.
- **OBE provides the basis for the allocation of resources to providers.** The contribution made by a course or subject to the overall learning outcomes can help to determine the allocation of time and resources to individual courses. In one medical school it was proposed that the duration of the obstetrics and gynaecology clerkship should be reduced significantly, given that competence in the delivery of a baby was no longer an undergraduate requirement. The proposal was quashed when the contributions of the clerkship to the school's overall learning outcomes were considered. Among other things, the course offered students valuable opportunities at the antenatal classes to understand health promotion and to appreciate clinical audit at the child and mother mortality conferences.
- **OBE ensures that the assessment is more valid.** OBE has particular significance for student assessment and the approach helps to ensure greater validity of the assessment. OBE is consistent with the move to more performance-based assessment and facilitates an assessment-to-a-standard approach where it is the standards students achieve that are important and not the time they take to achieve them.
- **OBE provides continuity across the continuum of medical education.** There is a need to have a more seamless continuum between the different phases of undergraduate, postgraduate and continuing medical education. OBE, by making explicit the outcomes for each of the phases or stages of education, provides a vocabulary to discuss the continuum and helps to encourage continuity between the phases.
- **OBE flags up problems in the curriculum.** Increasing attention has been focused on curriculum evaluation. Learning outcomes provide a yardstick against which a curriculum can be judged. A failure to achieve the agreed outcomes almost certainly identifies a problem with the curriculum.
- **OBE helps teachers to select the topics to be taught in a teaching session.** Consideration of the expected learning outcomes guides a teacher as to topics to be covered in a teaching session. Although it may be

tempting, teachers cannot simply address what is of interest to them. In the seventeenth century, the practice at Glasgow University was for teachers to do just that. They selected a book from their personal or the university's collection that interested them and read it to students in the lecture hall. The senior university position of 'reader' exists even today although the role is very different. The concept of a planned 'curriculum' with clarity of the outcomes expected was developed in response to student protests.

- **OBE enables curricula worldwide to be compared.** It is possible to compare education programmes in different countries using statements of outcomes. The Bologna process is concerned with harmonisation, not necessarily uniformity, in the higher education sector in Europe, and the Tuning Project has as its aim the establishment of a learning outcome framework for primary medical degree qualifications in Europe.

LEARNING OUTCOMES AND INSTRUCTIONAL OBJECTIVES

The concept of defining the learning outcomes for a programme of study is not new. The idea of instructional objectives promoted by Mager and others in the 1960s attracted much attention. Over the years, many teachers and curriculum planners have striven to specify the instructional objectives for their learning programmes. In practice, however, this initiative has had a disappointing impact on student learning and on the delivery of education programmes by teachers. While the concepts of learning outcomes and instructional objectives have much in common, there are significant differences:

- **Level and detail of specification.** Instructional objectives were specified in great detail as a bottom-up approach. The book of instructional objectives published by the Southern Illinois Medical School, for example, extended to more than 400 pages. In contrast learning outcomes, as we will see in the next chapter, represent a top-down approach and are specified as broader domains. This approach is more user-friendly and can more easily be adopted by teachers and students in their day-to-day activities.
- **Classification.** Instructional objectives were classified into knowledge, skills and attitudes categories. This ignores the complexities of medicine and the interaction of all three domains in medical practice. The outcome domains described in Chapter 7 are more holistic and resonate more closely with the work of a doctor.
- **Intent.** The language of instructional 'objectives' suggests aims or aspirations. An outcome-based education requires the teacher to take responsibility for the student achieving the outcomes expected.
- **Ownership of outcomes.** Instructional objectives were presented as a teacher-centred activity. In contrast, the specification of learning outcomes and their impact on the curriculum involves a partnership of students and teachers and encourages ownership of the process by the different stakeholders.

It should be acknowledged that in considerations of the product of learning, the terms 'aims', 'goals', 'objectives', 'competencies', 'abilities' and 'learning outcomes' are often used to describe the same thing. For practical purposes the terms 'learning outcomes' and 'competencies' can be regarded as interchangeable.

POTENTIAL PROBLEMS AND LIMITATIONS OF OBE

OBE as an educational approach in medical training is still in its infancy. While the approach offers many advantages it has also been criticised by some teachers and educators. Some concerns have been expressed about the approach. These include:

- a lack of research base that demonstrates the effectiveness of implementing an outcome-based education model
- demands imposed on teachers in implementing OBE, in specifying learning outcomes and in relating the outcomes to teaching and learning experiences and the assessment
- limitations placed on learning and the imposition of a rigid model on curriculum developers and teachers – concerns that the teacher will simply become an 'education technician'
- failure to address adequately in an outcome framework domains such as creativity, with the result that they will be ignored in an outcome-driven curriculum.

It is important to recognise, however, that these criticisms relate more to how OBE is implemented in practice rather than to the principle itself. The problems described can be avoided and the benefits of the approach are being increasingly documented. The benefits to be accrued significantly outweigh any disadvantages. OBE is not simply a passing fad and is now part of mainstream medical education.

REFLECT AND REACT

1. Learning outcomes can help you in your role as a medical teacher. Think about which of the reasons described above for implementing an OBE approach are relevant to your own teaching.
2. Are there learning outcomes specified for the course or training programme for which you are responsible? If so, are you familiar with them?

EXPLORING FURTHER

IF YOU HAVE A FEW HOURS

Harden, R.M., Crosby, J.R., Davis, M.H., 1999. Outcome-Based Education. AMEE Medical Education Guide No. 14 Part 2. An introduction to outcome-based education. Med. Teach. 21, 7–14.

Harden, R.M., 2002. Learning outcomes and instructional objectives: is there a difference. Med. Teach. 24, 151–155.

Hodges, B.D., 2009. Cracks and crevices: globalisation discourse and medical education. Med. Teach. 31, 910–917.

IF YOU HAVE MORE TIME

Burke, J. (Ed.), 1995. Outcomes, Learning and the Curriculum. Implications for NVQs, GNVQs and other qualifications. The Falmer Press, London.

Carraccio, C., Wolfsthal, S.D., Englander, R., et al., 2002. Shifting paradigms: from Flexner to competencies. Acad. Med. 77, 361–367.
This article reviews the literature on competency-based education in medicine.

Med. Teach, 2010, 32, 8, 629–691.
This issue of Medical Teacher is devoted to a discourse around competency-based medical education (CBME). The papers were authored by an international group of individuals with a special interest in CBME.

Morrison, G., Goldfarb, S., Lanken, P.N., 2010. Team training of medical students in the 21st century: Would Flexner approve? Acad. Med. 85, 254–259.
This article concludes that team-related competencies will have to be embedded into educational programmes for medical students.

Spady, W.G., 1994. Outcome-Based Education: Critical Issues and Answers. The American Association of School Administrators, Arlington, Virginia.
The classic text of Spady on the subject.

Specifying learning outcomes and competences

A range of approaches can be used to identify and define the expected learning outcomes.

SPECIFICATION OF LEARNING OUTCOMES

The previous chapter highlighted the benefits to be gained from the adoption in education of an outcome-based approach. The first step in implementing OBE is to define the learning outcomes required by the end of the training programme. This process is often initiated at a national level. In the UK the General Medical Council has set out in *Tomorrow's Doctors* their expectations for the learning outcomes of a graduate in a UK medical school. There are similar initiatives by the regulatory or accrediting bodies in the USA, Canada, Australia, the Netherlands, Saudi Arabia and many other countries. National examinations where they exist may also be viewed indirectly as statements of the expected learning outcomes.

While the learning outcomes will be to some extent specific to the context of a country, there are learning outcomes relating to what constitutes a good doctor that can be shared across geographical borders. In Europe, through a consultation process, generic and subject-specific competences expected of students at set points in the education programme are being identified. The International Institute for Medical Education in New York defined in terms of learning outcomes what they considered to be the 'global minimum essential requirements' for a doctor, whether in China or the USA.

The specification of learning outcomes is both a top-down and a bottom-up activity. A medical school can build on a national statement of learning outcomes with an expanded version reflecting the particular mission of the school. A community-oriented medical school or a school with the aim of qualifying the future researchers or leaders in medicine will reflect these orientations in its statement of learning outcomes. The Scottish medical schools, in 'The Scottish Doctor' report, specified the learning outcome domains subscribed to by all five Scottish schools. While the domains were agreed by all schools, more detailed learning outcome statements varied from school to school, mirroring the differences in the curriculum of the five schools.

Within each institution, detailed learning outcomes will be specified for each course and for each lecture or clinical training session within a course. These identify how each specific learning experience contributes to the exit learning outcomes for the school's education programme.

Just as with basic medical education programmes, OBE and the specification of learning outcomes are now features of training programmes for many specialties in medicine with the learning outcomes or competences agreed by the postgraduate training body or authority. In the USA the Accrediting Committee for Graduate Medical Education and, in Canada, the Royal College of Physicians and Surgeons have led the field.

LEARNING OUTCOMES AND THE CONTINUUM OF EDUCATION

For the most part, undergraduate, postgraduate and the continuing phases of education have been organised in separate silos each specifying independently their learning outcomes and the design of their learning programme. For almost 100 years there has been strong criticism of this separation or segregation. In 1932, the Final Report of the Commission of Medical Education in New York stated 'Artificial segregation of the basic medical course, the internship, the training of the specialist, or the continuation education of the general practitioner is very likely to create serious gaps in the education of physicians which should be avoided'. More recently, Cook, Irby and O'Brien, in *Educating Physicians*, a Carnegie follow-up to the 1910 Flexner Report in the USA, expressed concern that 'there is no single agency responsible for regulating and financing medical education; multiple agencies participate in this process and often hold conflicting expectations of programs and learners'. They highlighted the need for learning outcomes to bridge the continuum.

The development of an outcome-based approach offers a vocabulary that can facilitate discussion across the phases of education and hopefully this will serve as a catalyst for a more seamless continuum of medical education.

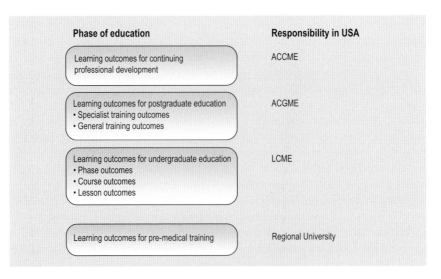

FIG 7.1 The learning outcomes and the different phases of education.

INVOLVEMENT OF STAKEHOLDERS

The specification of learning outcomes is a key step in the education process and the range of stakeholders should be involved. This may include:

- university staff
- hospital practitioners
- general practitioners
- recent graduates
- students
- other professions, e.g. nurses
- representatives of employers
- patients and representatives of patient groups
- the public.

The need for a wider consultation process is now accepted and is in keeping with a more patient-centred approach to care and a more general move to customer involvement in product development. Many of these stakeholders are now actively involved in curriculum committees. Such collaboration may help to align undergraduate, postgraduate and continuing education.

APPROACHES TO IDENTIFYING LEARNING OUTCOMES

The expected learning outcomes must match future expectations for the health care we want to see provided. Approaches that can be used to specify the expected learning outcomes include:

- the Delphi technique
- a critical incident survey
- studies of errors in practice
- task analysis
- a study of existing curricula and publications
- interviews with recent graduates.

THE DELPHI TECHNIQUE

The Delphi technique is a commonly used and successful way of identifying the expected learning outcomes. It relies on the judgement of an expert panel of 'wise men'. The 'experts', usually about 20 although it may be more, are required to define the learning outcomes that they consider necessary for medical practice. The circulated responses are then analysed, amended and added to or deleted where necessary by the participants, and the process is repeated until a consensus about a final list of learning outcomes is reached. The Delphi approach has been used to identify learning outcomes for basic medical education and for the training programmes in a range of medical specialties.

A CRITICAL INCIDENT SURVEY

Qualified individuals (not necessarily doctors) are asked to describe medical incidents that happened to them or that they observed which reflected good or bad medical practice. As the number of individually described incidents increases, the incidents tend to fall into natural clusters and the areas of essential competence in medicine begin to emerge. Blum and Fitzpatrick (1965) described a classic example of the use of this approach by the American Board of Orthopaedic Surgery. A variation of the critical incident survey is where those studied are regarded as 'star performers' and the features of a 'star performer' are identified.

STUDIES OF ERRORS IN PRACTICE

Errors occurring in medical practice may be an indicator of problems with the existing curriculum, and identification of these can contribute to the development of learning outcomes. This may be carried out in collaboration with medical defence or medical insurance bodies. The identification of a common pattern of errors in medical practice attributed to poor communication skills provided evidence that skills in communication should have a greater emphasis in the specification of learning outcomes and in the curriculum.

TASK ANALYSIS

Task analysis requires a researcher to follow a doctor on the job for a week or so and carefully list the tasks that the doctor carries out. The list provides a description of the activities that constitute the practice of medicine and can be the basis for the specification of the required learning outcomes. This approach is based on current practice and tells us what is done by a doctor today rather than what may be expected in the future. Nor does it give an indication necessarily of the competences or abilities required to undertake the tasks recorded.

STUDY OF EXISTING CURRICULA AND PUBLICATIONS

A useful starting off point for the determination of learning outcomes is a study of what is currently taught in a range of medical schools or postgraduate programmes, and the related outcomes. Analysis of the content of current textbooks and other publications may also be helpful.

INTERVIEWS WITH RECENT GRADUATES

Surveys of recent graduates can identify the strengths and weaknesses of the existing education programme and the stated learning outcomes. This can be done through interviews, focus groups or a questionnaire survey.

None of the techniques described is a panacea for specifying learning outcomes. It is likely that the development of an appropriate set of learning outcomes will require the use of a combination of different methods.

REFLECT AND REACT

1. If learning outcomes for your course have been produced, how were they derived and who was responsible?
2. If learning outcomes are not available, how would you set about producing them?

IF YOU HAVE A FEW HOURS

Blum, J.M., Fitzpatrick, R., 1965. Critical performance requirements for orthopaedic surgery: I. Method: II. Categories of performance (AIR-56-2/65-TR). American Institutes for Research, Pittsburgh, PA.
An early description in orthopaedics of the application of the critical incident approach.

Broomfield, D., Humphris, G.M., 2001. Using the Delphi technique to identify the cancer education requirements of general practitioners. Med. Educ. 35, 928–937.
An example of the use of the Delphi technique in continuing medical education.

Dunn, W.R., Hamilton, D.D., 1986. The critical incident technique – a brief guide. Med. Teach. 8, 207–215.
A useful review of Flanagan's critical incident technique.

Dunn, W.R., Hamilton, D.D., Harden, R.M., 1985. Techniques of identifying competencies needed of doctors. Med. Teach. 7, 15–25.
A description of the range of approaches that can be adopted in the specification of learning outcomes

General Medical Council, 2009. Tomorrow's Doctors. General Medical Council, London.
Outcomes for undergraduate medical education.

Laidlaw, J.M., Harden, R.M., Morris, A.M., 1995. Needs assessment and the development of an educational programme on malignant melanoma for general practitioners. Med. Teach. 17, 79–87.
A description of how the learning needs were addressed for a continuing education programme for general practitioners.

Paterson, A., Hesketh, E.A., Macpherson, S.G., Harden, R.M., 2004. Exit learning outcomes for the PRHO year: an evidence base for informed decisions. Med. Educ. 38, 67–80.
An example of the use of the Delphi process in the establishment of learning outcomes.

Describing and communicating the learning outcomes

Different frameworks or models can be used to categorise and communicate learning outcomes.

LEARNING FRAMEWORKS

Learning outcomes are structured round a number of domains – usually no more than 12. Each domain represents a category of learning outcomes, for example clinical skills. Learning outcomes are then specified for each of the domains.

Several frameworks or models for grouping learning outcomes have been described. Not surprisingly the different frameworks, while having significant differences, have much in common. Some of the most widely used frameworks are described below.

THE DUNDEE THREE-CIRCLE OUTCOME MODEL AND 'THE SCOTTISH DOCTOR' FRAMEWORK

This framework is based on 12 domains. It is different from other frameworks in that the domains are incorporated in a three-circle model that emphasises the relationship between the different domains (Fig. 8.1). We have looked in Chapter 5 at a similar model for describing the good teacher.

The *inner circle* represents the technical skills of the doctor or what the doctor is able to do – 'doing the right thing'. It includes seven domains:

1. clinical skills
2. practical procedures
3. patient investigations
4. patient management
5. health promotion and disease prevention
6. communication
7. information handling skills.

The *middle circle* represents the way the doctor approaches the tasks in the inner circle –'doing the thing right':

8. understanding of social, basic and clinical sciences
9. appropriate attitudes and ethical understanding
10. decision making skills and clinical judgement.

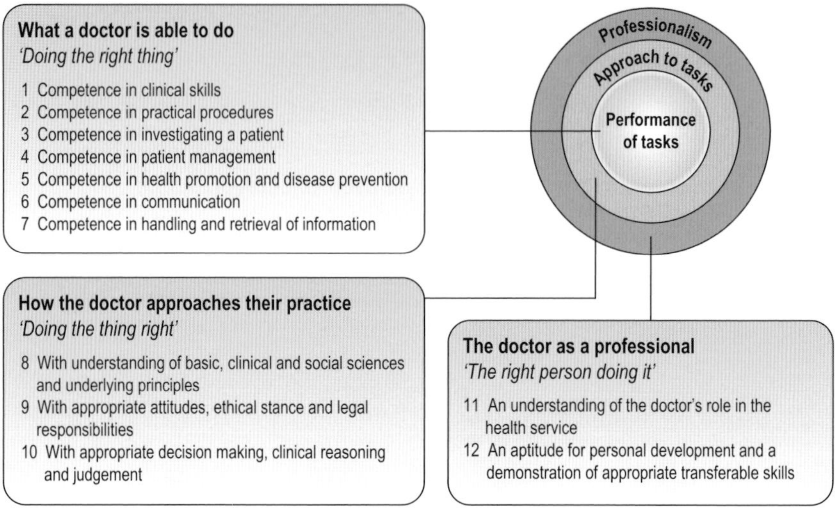

FIG 8.1 The three-circle model for learning outcomes incorporating 12 domains.

The *outer circle* represents the development of the personal attributes of the individual – 'the right person doing it':

11. the role of the doctor.
12. personal development.

This model is described in more detail in Appendix 6.

The three-circle model with the 12 outcome domains has been adopted in 'The Scottish Doctor' as a description of the abilities of medical graduates from the five Scottish Medical Schools. The approach has also been used in other countries.

THE CANMEDS PHYSICIAN COMPETENCY FRAMEWORK

The Royal College of Physicians and Surgeons of Canada developed a framework built round seven physician roles. These make explicit the abilities of the highly skilled physician. The roles are:

1. Medical expert: applying knowledge skills and attitudes to patient care.
2. Communicator: communicating effectively with patients, families, colleagues and other professionals.
3. Collaborator: working effectively within a healthcare team.
4. Health advocate: advancing the health and well-being of patients and populations.
5. Manager: participating effectively in the organisation of the healthcare system.
6. Scholar: committing to reflective learning as well as to the creation, dissemination and application of medical knowledge.
7. Professional: committing to ethical practice and high personal standard of behaviour.

Figure 8.2 illustrates the elements and the interconnections of the roles.

The CanMEDS competency framework has been used in postgraduate and continuing education in Canada and worldwide and has also been adopted for use in undergraduate education.

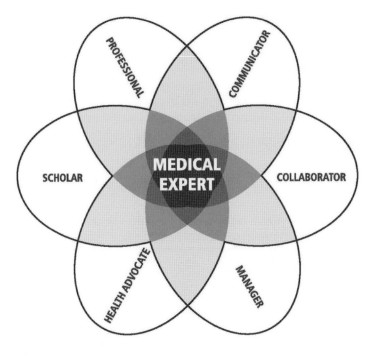

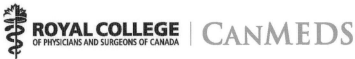

FIG 8.2 The CanMEDS Roles Framework. *Adapted from the CanMEDS Physician Competency Diagram with permission of the Royal College of Physicians and Surgeons of Canada. Copyright ©2009.*

THE ACCREDITATION COUNCIL FOR GRADUATE MEDICAL EDUCATION (ACGME)

The Accreditation Council for Graduate Medical Education in the USA developed a model based on six competency domains closely aligned with healthcare quality aims. These were:

1. patient care
2. medical knowledge
3. practice-based learning and improvement
4. inter-personal and communication skills
5. professionalism
6. systems-based practice.

The ACGME competencies are used both internationally and in US postgraduate medical education programmes to foster and assess resident physicians' development in the six domains. They have also been adopted in undergraduate education.

THE BROWN ABILITIES

Brown University in the USA was one of the first medical schools to adopt an outcome-based approach to education. A series of nine abilities was developed from the tasks that are expected of physicians practising in the twenty-first century and the attributes needed to perform the tasks competently. The Brown description of learning outcomes is of interest in that it describes for each of the nine abilities observable behaviours that students must demonstrate at the beginning, intermediate and advanced levels of their training.

The nine abilities identified to describe a successful doctor are:

1. effective communication
2. basic clinical skills
3. using basic science in the practice of medicine
4. diagnosis, management and prevention of disease
5. lifelong learning
6. self-awareness, self-care and personal growth
7. the social and community context of health care
8. moral reasoning and clinical ethics
9. problem solving.

GLOBAL MINIMUM ESSENTIAL REQUIREMENTS (GMER)

The Institute for International Medical Education of the China Medical Board in New York, working with an international network of experts in medical education, developed the global minimum essential requirements (GMER) as a set of learning outcomes that highlight the competencies expected of graduates from medical schools in countries throughout the world.

The seven domains are:

1. professional values, attitudes, behaviour and ethics
2. scientific foundation of medicine
3. clinical skills
4. communication skills
5. population health and health systems
6. management of information
7. critical thinking and research.

CRITERIA FOR A LEARNING OUTCOME FRAMEWORK

A learning outcome framework should meet the following criteria:

- The key domains should reflect the vision and mission of the institution as perceived by the various stakeholders including the public. They should reflect clearly, with an appropriate sense of values, what is expected of a doctor.
- The domains should be defined at an appropriate level of generality. The number of domains should be small enough to be manageable but large enough to distinguish the different aspects of competence.
- The framework should provide a holistic and integrated view of medical practice and indicate the relationship between the different outcome domains.

- The framework should assist with the development of 'enabling' outcomes for each of the key domains specified.
- The framework should be clear and unambiguous. It should be user-friendly, intuitive and easy to use.

REFLECT AND REACT

1. Agreement may already have been reached regarding the outcome framework that is used in your situation. If not, you can develop your own framework or select and adapt an existing framework. The latter approach has obvious advantages.
2. Are teachers and students familiar with the details of the framework and how the elements of the education programme for which you have a responsibility relate to the overall outcome framework?

EXPLORING FURTHER

IF YOU HAVE A FEW HOURS

2007. Med. Teach. 29 (7).
This issue of the journal has as its theme outcome-based education. It includes a series of articles describing the different OBE frameworks.

IF YOU HAVE MORE TIME

The CanMEDS, 2005. Physician Competency Framework. Better Standards. Better Physicians. Better Care. In: Frank, J.R. (Ed.), The Royal College of Physicians and Surgeons of Canada, Ottawa.

An introduction to the CanMeds framework with a more detailed description of the CanMeds roles.
Scottish Deans' Medical Education Group, 2008. The Scottish Doctor. Learning outcomes for the Medical Undergraduate in Scotland; A Foundation for Competent and Reflective Practitioners. The Association for Medical Education in Europe (AMEE), Dundee.
A description of the 12 outcome domains subdivided into a more detailed set of learning outcomes.

Implementing an outcome-based approach in practice

Outcome-based education requires two things. The learning outcomes need to be identified and specified. Decisions about the curriculum must be based on the specified outcomes.

THE OSTRICHES, THE PEACOCKS AND THE BEAVERS

Outcome-based education, as discussed in Chapter 6, is about more than defining and publishing a set of learning outcomes that must be achieved before the end of the course. OBE is characterised by a curriculum with the learning strategies and learning opportunities designed to ensure that students achieve the learning outcomes specified and with an assessment process matched to the learning outcomes. Individual students are assessed to ensure that they achieve the outcomes. Remediation and enrichment for students is provided as appropriate.

Teachers react differently when it comes to implementing OBE. Some consider OBE to be a passing fad and make no effort to either prepare learning outcomes or incorporate them into their teaching. They bury their heads in the sand and can be likened to ostriches (Harden 2007). Then there are teachers who work hard producing a set or list of learning outcomes that is prominently displayed for visitors or programme assessors – the peacocks. Unfortunately they do not make use of the learning outcomes in their teaching, so their efforts are to no avail. The teachers who do successfully implement an OBE approach are those who believe that OBE is the way to design, deliver and document instruction and work hard to make this happen – the beavers.

PLANNING AN OBE PROGRAMME

An OBE curriculum starts with the question – what are the expected learning outcomes to be achieved by the end of the programme and what capabilities should the graduate have as a practising doctor? An outcome framework is used, as described in Chapter 8, to describe the broad performance capabilities. These in turn are specified in more detail. For example, in the broad domain of patient management a more detailed set of learning outcomes includes surgery, drugs, physiotherapy, social dimensions and alternative therapies.

After the exit learning outcomes are defined, working backwards, outcomes are specified for each of the courses or attachments in the curriculum. These will identify how the course contributes overall to the school's exit learning outcomes. For example the learning outcomes achieved in an anatomy course may go beyond the mastery and understanding of anatomy and, as identified by Pawlina in the Mayo Clinic, can include communication skills and teamwork. The outcomes are specified further for each of the learning experiences in a course or attachment, for example a lecture, a clinical session or a practical experience. It is helpful to produce a grid or blueprint that relates each of the learning experiences to the learning outcomes for the course. A similar grid should be produced that relates the assessment to the learning outcomes. The clearer the definition of learning outcomes, the more effectively can student assessment be planned. The appropriate tools are selected according to the outcomes to be assessed. An assessment profile can be produced for each student that highlights the outcomes that have been achieved and those that have not.

STUDENT PROGRESSION IN AN OBE CURRICULUM

It is recognised that there are legitimate differences as to the manner and rate at which students progress to the exit learning outcomes. Some students, for example, may acquire the necessary communication skills more quickly than others. Students' achievements of the learning outcomes can be used to monitor and plan for their progression through the curriculum. Mastery of an outcome to a specified standard may be a requirement before the student is allowed to progress from one part of the medical course to the next. A student may be required to have a certain mastery not only of basic sciences but of communication skills before proceeding to clinical studies in the later years of the course. Progression can also be charted across the continuum of education from undergraduate through postgraduate to continuing education.

Four dimensions can be considered with regard to students' achievements of learning outcomes and their progression through the course and these are described in Chapter 12.

AN OBE IMPLEMENTATION INVENTORY

An OBE implementation inventory can be used to describe a school's or postgraduate body's level of adoption of an OBE approach in their education programme. This can be rated on a five-point scale in each of nine dimensions as shown in Figure 9.1:

1. The extent to which there is a clear and unambiguous statement of the learning outcomes expected.
2. Whether staff and students in an institution are made aware of and are familiar with the outcome statements.
3. The extent to which the educational strategies adopted, such as problem-based learning, community-based learning or inter-professional learning, reflect the learning outcomes. The ability to work as a member of a team alongside other healthcare professionals, for example, can be facilitated through inter-professional learning experiences.

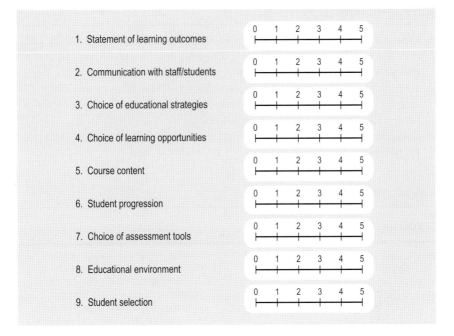

FIG 9.1 OBE implementation profile.

4. The matching of the learning opportunities selected with the learning outcomes. Almost certainly this will require the use of a range of teaching and learning methods.

5. A significant problem facing medical education is the rapid expansion of knowledge with the associated danger of information overload and curriculum congestion. Consideration of the learning outcomes can help to determine what content should be covered in the curriculum.

6. The students' achievements of the learning outcomes can be used to assess their progression through the curriculum and to determine whether they are able to proceed to the next stage.

7. The learning outcomes are important in relation to assessment. Serious problems arise when there is a mismatch between the learning outcomes, the learning experiences and the student assessment.

8. In planning an education programme, increased attention is being paid to the educational environment. This is described in Chapter 18. In OBE, the learning outcomes specified can indicate what should be a desirable learning environment. For example, a learning outcome addressing teamwork skills should suggest the need for an educational environment that supports collaborative working rather than the more typical environment where competition is rewarded.

9. The final dimension in the inventory relates to the selection of students. It can be argued that with an OBE approach, the exit learning outcomes should be reflected in the admission criteria for students. Students should be assessed on the entry-level requirements for each of the outcome domains such as communication skills, problem solving and attitudes.

REFLECT AND REACT

1. Where on the OBE inventory does your school or postgraduate body lie? Are you well on the way to an outcome-based approach or are you still at the early stages of implementation?
2. Have you clearly identified outcomes for your own areas of teaching responsibility and is it clear how these contribute to the overall outcomes for the training or education programme?
3. Consider how you use learning outcomes to monitor and guide students' progression.

EXPLORING FURTHER

IF YOU HAVE A FEW HOURS

Harden, R.M., 2007a. Outcome-based education – the ostrich, the peacock and the beaver. Med. Teach. 29, 666–671.
A description of the OBE implementation inventory and how it helps teachers, schools and education bodies to create a profile of the extent to which OBE has been implemented in the institution.

Harden, R.M., 2007b. Learning outcomes as a tool to assess progression. Med. Teach. 29, 678–682.
A description of how students progress to the achievement of the learning outcomes.

IF YOU HAVE MORE TIME

Burke, J. (Ed.), 1995. Outcomes, Learning and the Curriculum. Implications for NVQs, GNVQs and other qualifications. The Falmer Press, London.

A general early description of the curricular consequences of an outcome-based approach to education and training more generally.

Holmboe, E.S., Ward, D.S., Reznick, R.K., et al., 2011. Faculty development in assessment: the missing link in competency-based medical education. Acad. Med. 86, 460–467.
The authors argue that medical education needs an international initiative of faculty development around competency-based medical education.

SECTION 3
ORGANISING THE LEARNING PROGRAMME

'Teachers don't merely deliver the curriculum. They develop, define it and interpret it too.'
Michael Fullan and Andrew Hargreaves. *Understanding Teacher Development*, 1994

OVERVIEW

Planning and implementing a curriculum presents a significant challenge.

Chapter 10 What constitutes a curriculum?
The curriculum is more than just a syllabus or timetable. It embraces all of the learning opportunities both formal and informal.

Chapter 11 Ten questions to ask when planning a curriculum
Planning and implementing a curriculum requires careful attention to detail. Ten questions provide a useful checklist.

Chapter 12 Sequencing the content and the spiral curriculum
Sequencing the content can prove complex. Some approaches may be more effective than others in helping the learner to achieve the expected learning outcomes.

Chapter 13 Adopting a student-centred approach
The role of the teacher has to change when we empower students to take more responsibility for their own learning.

Chapter 14 Building learning around problems and clinical presentations
A clinical problem or task undertaken by a healthcare professional can serve as the basis for learning. The student is motivated by the more authentic learning experience.

Chapter 15 Using an integrated and inter-professional approach
An integrated curriculum, bringing together different disciplines, offers major advantages. There are also benefits from sharing learning experiences with different professions.

Chapter 16 Making the apprenticeship model and work-based learning more effective
There is no better way to learn than from work-related experience. This requires careful monitoring and supervision.

Chapter 17 Building options into a core curriculum

Alongside a core curriculum that provides the necessary breadth of study, options and electives provide an opportunity for students to study selected topics in more depth.

Chapter 18 Recognising the importance of the education environment

This neglected area is now recognised as being a substantial and very real element that influences students' learning. Tools are available to assess the education environment.

Chapter 19 Mapping the curriculum

A clear picture of how learning outcomes, teaching methods and student assessment link together is crucial not only for the teacher but also for the student. A curriculum map is needed.

What constitutes a curriculum?

The curriculum is more than just a syllabus or timetable. It embraces all of the learning opportunities both formal and informal.

THE CONCEPT OF A CURRICULUM

The curriculum was equated in the past with the syllabus and the timetable. A curriculum document included a statement about content, the subjects covered and the courses that students should attend. This concept of a curriculum has been widened to include:

- the learning outcomes
- the teaching and learning methods
- the educational strategies
- the context for the learning
- the learning environment
- the assessment procedures.

Each of these aspects of a curriculum is explored in more detail in Chapter 11. A curriculum can be thought of as made up of all the experiences learners have that enable them to achieve the specified learning outcomes (Grant 2010).

APPROACHES TO THE CURRICULUM

All of the above elements are important and need to be taken into consideration when a curriculum is planned. Particular attention is paid sometimes to one aspect:

- **The architect approach.** Just as in architecture, work starts here with a full specification of what is to be produced. The focus for curriculum planning is on a detailed statement of the aims of the medical school and the expected learning outcomes.
- **The mechanic approach.** The car mechanic is concerned with the type of engine rather than the direction in which the car has to travel. The focus for the curriculum planning is on the teaching approaches and the learning opportunities created.
- **The cookbook approach.** Just as in cookbook recipes with lists and quantities of the ingredients for the cakes and other dishes, a detailed list is made of all the contents that have to go in to the curriculum.

- **The railway approach.** The railway timetable comprises the routes and times when trains arrive and depart at different stations. In the railway approach the emphasis is on the students' timetable and their activities and venues at each hour of the day.
- **The religious approach.** Just as in religion where there is a principle or system of tenets held with devotion, so those responsible for planning the curriculum hold some value or curriculum strategy, such as problem-based learning, to be of supreme importance.
- **The detective approach.** The emphasis is on identifying problems in relation to the existing curriculum just as the detective has to assess the evidence and diagnose a problem at the scene of a crime.
- **The bureaucratic approach.** Here a major factor is the rules and regulations, sometimes imposed from outside, that govern an institution or school and its curriculum.
- **The magician approach.** In this approach a curriculum appears just like a magician produces a rabbit out of a hat. It is not clear how the curriculum has been derived or who has been responsible for its production.

While these hopefully represent caricatures of curriculum planning they unfortunately occasionally represent what happens in practice. Today, in both undergraduate and postgraduate education we should be far removed from 'a magician approach' to curriculum planning. As described in the next chapters, development of a curriculum is a systematic process that involves a series of planned steps with attention paid to all of the elements. The curriculum is seen as an expression of intentions, mechanisms and context of the education programme that requires input from all of the stakeholders including teachers, students, administrators, employers, the government and the wider public.

THE PLANNED, THE DELIVERED AND THE LEARNED CURRICULUM

A distinction can be made between:

- The 'planned' curriculum that is documented and agreed by the curriculum planners and teachers and embodies their intentions and aspirations – the curriculum on paper.

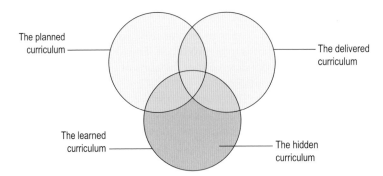

FIG 10.1 The 'planned', the 'delivered' and the 'learned' curriculum.

- The 'actual' or 'delivered' curriculum, which is the reality of the students' or trainees' experiences and what is delivered or happens in practice – the curriculum in action.
- The 'learned curriculum', which represents the students' knowledge, skills and attitudes that result from their learning experience.

A mismatch between the 'planned' and the 'delivered' curriculum may be due to a teacher's lack of familiarity or acceptance of the specified curriculum, or to the fact that the realities of any course will never fully match the hopes and intentions of the planners. Occasionally the problem may arise from a deliberate intent by teachers to emphasise what they think is important and should be taught rather than what is specified in the curriculum. Teachers can sabotage a curriculum. They need to be committed to it and accept the underlying principles. It is the teacher's responsibility to keep any differences between the planned and delivered curriculum to a minimum. Where there are significant differences, the reason for these should be analysed and action taken as necessary. Logistical problems, problems with students or trainees or inherent issues with the planned curriculum should be addressed.

Part of the 'learned curriculum' is the 'hidden curriculum'. This can be thought of as the outcomes that are not part of the explicit intentions of those planning a curriculum. These may be knowledge and skills but more importantly may be attitudes and beliefs. The formal curriculum is described in the course documents, prospectus and study guides. The hidden or unofficial curriculum is determined by the educational environment and relates to the students' experiences as described in Chapter 18. There may be conflict, particularly in relation to ethical decisions, between the hidden curriculum and what they are taught in the formal curriculum.

REFLECT AND REACT

1. How familiar are you with the details of your students' curriculum? Do you contribute to the curriculum's on-going evolution?
2. How would you characterise the approach adopted in the development of the curriculum?
3. How important in your context is the 'hidden curriculum' and how closely aligned are the planned and the delivered curriculum?

EXPLORING FURTHER

IF YOU HAVE A FEW HOURS

Davis, M.H., Harden, R.M., 2003. Planning and implementing an undergraduate medical curriculum: the lessons learned. Med. Teach. 25, 596–608.
A description of the approach to curriculum development adopted in one medical school.

Grant, J., 2010. Principles of curriculum design. In: Swanwick, T. (Ed.), Understanding Medical Education: Evidence, Theory and Practice. Wiley-Blackwell, Chichester.

Hafferty, F.W., Castellani, B., 2009. The hidden curriculum. A theory of medical education. In: Brosnan, C., Turner, B.S. (Eds.), Handbook of the Sociology of Medical Education. Routledge, London, pp. 15–35.
An exploration of the hidden curriculum. The development of the concept can be attributed to Hafferty.

Harden, R.M., 1986. Approaches to curriculum planning. Med. Educ. 20, 458–466.
An account of the different approaches to curriculum planning introduced in this chapter.

IF YOU HAVE MORE TIME

Fish, D., Coles, C., 2005. Developing a Curriculum for Practice. Medical Education. Open University Press, Maidenhead.
An account of curriculum development in medical education.

Kelly, A.V., 2004. The Curriculum, Theory and Practice, fifth ed. Sage Publications, London.
A classic book on the curriculum. Although more focused on the curriculum in schools, the ideas and concepts have relevance to medical education.

Ten questions to ask when planning a curriculum

Planning and implementing a curriculum requires careful attention to detail. Ten questions provide a useful checklist.

Curriculum development is a serious business that requires careful consideration and planning. In this chapter we highlight ten questions that need to be addressed:

1. What are the needs to be met by the training programme?
2. What are the expected learning outcomes?
3. What content should be included?
4. How should the content be organised?
5. What educational strategies should be adopted?
6. What teaching methods should be used?
7. How should assessment be carried out?
8. How should details of the curriculum be communicated?
9. What educational environment or climate should be fostered?
10. How should the process be managed?

WHAT ARE THE NEEDS TO BE MET BY THE TRAINING PROGRAMME?

The needs to be met by a curriculum are often ignored or taken for granted. There are merits in stepping back and considering these. More attention needs to be paid to the mission of a medical school with regards to its social accountability and the extent to which it trains doctors to work in the community it serves.

The traditional curriculum may not train doctors who are motivated and equipped to work in rural areas. In Australia, Canada and other countries where this is seen as a healthcare need, significant resources have been allocated to support curricula and training facilities with an emphasis on medical practice in rural settings. Matching the education programme to healthcare needs is important and of concern not just for the medical school but also for the range of stakeholders including the government, the public at large and other healthcare professions. The role of the doctor and how he or she fits into the healthcare team should be pivotal in the creation of a medical programme.

Another issue that merits more consideration is the response by medical schools to globalisation and the international dimensions of medical practice. Schools need to recognise the greater mobility in the medical workforce and the importance of graduating doctors who have the skills necessary as global citizens.

WHAT ARE THE EXPECTED LEARNING OUTCOMES?

Key to a curriculum are the learning outcomes expected of the learner. We highlighted in Section 2 the importance of learning outcomes and the move away from an emphasis on the *education process* to an outcome-based education model where the emphasis is on *the product.* We looked at how learning outcomes can be expressed and communicated relating to technical competencies and clinical skills; approaches to practice embracing an understanding of the basic sciences, appropriate attitudes and decision-making strategies; and personal development and professionalism. Decisions about the learning outcomes should inform the answers to the questions that follow.

WHAT CONTENT SHOULD BE INCLUDED?

With the rapid expansion of medical and scientific knowledge and the development of new specialties, information overload is now a major problem facing medical education. While the content has expanded, the time available in the curriculum has remained relatively constant. Decisions need to be taken regarding what is to be included in the core curriculum and what is omitted. There has been considerable debate about the coverage in the undergraduate curriculum of anatomy and other basic sciences and whether it is possible to provide an overview and necessary understanding without embracing the detailed basic science and anatomical knowledge covered in the past.

There will be an agreed core content which has to be mastered by all students, with opportunities to study other subjects through electives or student-selected courses, as described in Chapter 17.

Doctors can now readily access information when they require it, through the internet and other sources. The core content curriculum must provide students with the vocabulary, understanding and skills necessary to identify and interpret this information.

HOW SHOULD THE CONTENT BE ORGANISED?

With the learning outcomes and the content determined, the next step is to consider how the curriculum should be organised and the content sequenced. The traditional approach in medical education has been to introduce students first to the basic medical sciences and normal function, structure and behaviour of the human body. As students progressed through the curriculum to the later years, the focus was on abnormal function and the development of clinical skills. Later, students developed their clinical competence on the job as they managed patients. This sequence, while having much to commend it, has disadvantages. The relevance of the content is not obvious to the student and, as we discuss in Chapter 2, as a consequence the learning may be less effective. How content can be arranged and sequenced in a way that leads to more effective and efficient learning as students progress through their training is important and is covered in Chapter 12.

WHAT EDUCATIONAL STRATEGIES SHOULD BE ADOPTED?

Educational strategies may be seen as the key element in a curriculum with the curriculum labelled in terms of the educational strategy, e.g. a 'problem-based curriculum' and 'a community orientated curriculum'. The SPICES model for curriculum planning identifies six educational approaches and presents each on a continuum (Fig. 11.1).

STUDENT-CENTRED/TEACHER-CENTRED

There has been a significant move towards a more student-centred approach in the curriculum, as described in Chapter 13, with students given more responsibility for their own learning. It is what students learn that matters and not what teachers teach. Teachers are being challenged and programmes scrutinised to establish whether they are meeting the needs of individual students in terms of content, approaches to learning and time taken to complete.

PROBLEM-BASED/INFORMATION-ORIENTATED

A problem-based approach to learning has been adopted in a number of schools over the past two decades. The starting-off point and the focus for the learning is a clinical problem. It is what the students need to know to understand the problem that drives their activities. This topic is discussed further in Chapter 14. Task-based learning is described as a variation of problem-based learning.

S	Student-centred ....Teacher-centred
P	Problem-based ....Information-oriented
I	Integrated or inter-professional....................................Discipline-based
C	Community-based ....Hospital-based
E	Elective-driven ....Uniform
S	Systematic..Opportunistic

FIG 11.1 The SPICES model of educational strategies.

INTEGRATED/DISCIPLINE-BASED

There has been a significant move away from curricula based on courses that relate to individual subjects or disciplines such as anatomy, surgery and pathology, to courses integrated around body systems such as the cardiovascular system. There is also a move towards a greater integration between the basic medical sciences and clinical subjects. An inter-professional approach where different professions share, to a greater or lesser extent, their learning experiences is being explored and implemented in some education programmes. This makes sense given the need for students to develop teamwork skills. Integration and inter-professional education is explored further in Chapter 15.

COMMUNITY BASED/HOSPITAL BASED

There has been a move away from a curriculum that provides only a hospital-based setting for students to gain their experience. More attractive is a curriculum that, in addition, offers experience in a community setting. This is covered in Chapter 16.

ELECTIVE/UNIFORM

A curriculum should include both core elements common to all students, and electives or student-selected components. Such options provide students with a choice of topics for their study. The concept of a core curriculum with options is addressed in Chapter 17.

SYSTEMATIC (PLANNED)/APPRENTICESHIP (OPPORTUNISTIC)

In a systematic curriculum, there is a clear statement of the learning outcomes and teaching, learning and assessment is planned and related to the outcomes. This is in contrast to an apprenticeship or opportunistic model where lecturers address whatever topic is of interest to them and students' experiences attached to a clinical unit depend on the patients they see as they present during the attachment.

Where an education programme is located on each of these six dimensions is key to curriculum planning and likely to be specific for the institution. Almost certainly the position taken will not be at the extreme ends of the continua. The SPICES model can be used also for curriculum evaluation with the current position on the continua compared with the desired or optimum position for the school.

WHAT TEACHING METHODS SHOULD BE USED?

In the medical curriculum, traditional teaching approaches include lectures, small group activities and clinical clerkships together with textbooks and other learning resources. All of these have a role to play. A more recent feature is the adoption of new learning technologies including e-learning and the use of simulators perhaps located in a clinical skills centre.

Student support for and learning from each other has always been a feature of the education process. A more recent development has been peer-assisted learning where students are formally involved in the education of their peers or more junior students.

A description of traditional approaches and the introduction of exciting newer methods is provided in Section 4.

HOW SHOULD ASSESSMENT BE CARRIED OUT?

A key element in the curriculum and one that significantly influences students' behaviour is assessment. It is essential that assessment matches closely the expected learning outcomes. Decisions have to be taken about the overall assessment strategy and the appropriate instruments to be adopted with this in mind. The objective structured clinical examination (OSCE) and assessment portfolios have been introduced to meet the need for more authentic and performance assessment instruments. Work-based assessment is growing in popularity particularly in postgraduate education. Section 5 describes established and newer approaches to assessment and the key issues that have to be addressed when an assessment programme is planned.

HOW SHOULD DETAILS OF THE CURRICULUM BE COMMUNICATED?

With the increased sophistication of the undergraduate and postgraduate curriculum and the use of strategies such as problem-based learning and integration, students and trainees require assistance with understanding:

- what is expected of them
- the learning opportunities available
- how to make best use of the learning opportunities
- their progress through the curriculum.

Teachers and trainers, too, may have difficulty in grasping their role in the process and in appreciating what is expected of their students in the phase of the programme for which they have responsibility.

If the curriculum is to succeed, effective communication about the curriculum and what is expected of teachers and students is necessary. This can be achieved through clear documentation and meetings with staff and students. The curriculum document should include:

- a clear statement and explanation of the expected learning outcomes
- a series of blueprints relating the learning outcomes to the available learning opportunities, the phases of the curriculum and the assessment
- a curriculum map, as described in Chapter 19, that shows the relationship between the different elements in the curriculum.

WHAT EDUCATIONAL ENVIRONMENT OR CLIMATE SHOULD BE FOSTERED?

Important, but often ignored in the consideration of the curriculum, is the educational climate or environment. This is the overall atmosphere of the school or wherever learning is taking place. It embraces, for example, the extent to

Ten questions to ask when planning a curriculum

which students feel they are studying in a supportive or threatening environment and whether the environment encourages teamwork and collaboration, appropriate professional behaviour, and creativity. A number of instruments are available that allow the educational environment to be measured. This topic is discussed in Chapter 18.

HOW SHOULD THE PROCESS BE MANAGED?

It should be obvious by now that the development and management of a curriculum is a substantial activity that requires careful planning and allocation of time and resources. Most medical schools and postgraduate bodies have recognised this and have set up committees charged with responsibility for the curriculum. A curriculum planning committee should represent all the stakeholders. Both hospital- and community-based interests should be represented, and junior and senior staff and students should be included.

Individual members of staff should be allocated responsibility for implementing the different aspects of the programme including:

- the coordination of each phase in the curriculum
- the organisation and delivery of each course
- the management of electives and options
- student assessment
- support for students including students with difficulties
- computer and information technology
- a clinical skills centre and the use of simulators and simulated patients.

It is important that staff who contribute to the education programme are recognised and rewarded for their efforts. This should include promotion on the basis of their contribution to teaching and the scholarship of education.

Educational programmes that are most successful have strong leadership from deans or clinical directors with support given by them for changes and innovations in the curriculum.

REFLECT AND REACT

1. Think about the ten questions as they relate to your own teaching situation. You may not be a member of a curriculum committee or directly involved with curriculum planning, but as a stakeholder you have an important role to play and will be able to discharge your responsibilities more effectively if you have an understanding of the issues involved.
2. Think about the educational strategies for the educational programme with which you are involved. Where do you lie on the SPICES continuum and where would you like to be?

IF YOU HAVE A FEW HOURS

Harden, R.M., 1986. Ten questions to ask when planning a course or curriculum. Med. Educ. 20, 356–365.
A description of the ten questions to be asked when planning a curriculum.

Harden, R.M., Sowden, S., Dunn, W.R., 1984. Some educational strategies in curriculum development: the SPICES model. ASME Medical Education Booklet No. 18. Med. Educ. 18, 284–297.
A description of the SPICES model and how it can be used in curriculum planning and evaluation.

IF YOU HAVE MORE TIME

Fleiszer, D.M., Posel, N.H., 2003. Development of an undergraduate medical curriculum: the McGill experience. Acad. Med. 78, 265–269.
A useful case study.

Grant, J., 2010. Principles of curriculum design. In: Swanwick, T. (Ed.), Understanding Medical Education: Evidence, Theory and Practice. Wiley-Blackwell, Chichester.
A description of the steps in curriculum design.

Kern, D.E., Thomas, P.A., Howard, D.M., Bass, E.B., 2011. Curriculum Development for Medical Education. A Six-Step Approach. The Johns Hopkins University Press, Baltimore and London.
A description of a six-step approach to curriculum development based on the author's experience at The Johns Hopkins School of Medicine.

Sequencing the content and the spiral curriculum

Sequencing the content can prove complex. Some approaches may be more effective than others in helping the learner to achieve the expected learning outcomes.

THE IMPORTANCE OF SEQUENCING

Much attention has been paid to the different elements that comprise the medical curriculum – the learning outcomes, the content of the curriculum, teaching and learning methods, educational strategies and assessment. Less attention has been paid to the overall organisation and sequence of learning within the curriculum. It is important to consider the big picture of the curriculum and how courses are sequenced as well as which courses are included. Sequencing of courses in the curriculum involves:

- **The arrangement of courses in a specific order.** Prerequisites for one course may include the learning outcomes achieved in an earlier course. The order of courses can help students to organise meaningful patterns in the vast amount of content knowledge so that they are less likely to forget what they have learned and are able to apply knowledge to new problems or unfamiliar contexts. The earlier introduction in the curriculum of clinical experiences provides students with a context for their learning.
- **Establishing the connectivity and interdependence of courses.** Students should be assisted in identifying connections between what they are currently learning, what they have previously learned, and what they have still to learn.

GUIDELINES FOR SEQUENCING

Of prime consideration in the sequencing of courses are:

- **The prerequisites.** The knowledge or skills that the students need before entering the course.
- **The course content.** What the students are required to study to master the expected learning outcomes.
- **Application of the competencies gained.** Students' continued learning following the course.

73

Curriculum sequencing involves managing the students' learning route in a way that makes it easier for them to achieve the learning outcomes. This may involve moving from:

- the simple to the complex
- general information or principles to a more detailed consideration
- basic principles to applications in practice.

This does not necessarily represent the optimum learning sequence. If students fail to see the relevance of courses to their ultimate goals they may lack motivation and learning may be ineffective. This is one reason for the move to introduce clinical courses and experiences earlier in the curriculum.

In some situations the sequencing of courses may be influenced by logistics. In clinical rotations, for instance, students may undertake clinical specialty attachments in different sequences, not all being optimal.

There is no doubt that issues relating to sequencing are complex, but here are two thoughts that merit consideration when the sequence of subjects in a curriculum is being determined:

1. The logical ordering of content that is already obvious to a subject specialist is not necessarily the most appropriate way for a student to learn the subject.
2. The prime aim in ordering the content of a course is to help students to learn most effectively. The introduction of students to patients in the early years of the course leads to better learning of the basic medical sciences.

EARLY CLINICAL EXPERIENCE

An important issue in sequencing relates to the relationship between the basic sciences and the clinical subjects. In the traditional undergraduate curriculum it was assumed that students should first acquire an understanding of the structure and function of the body before they considered pathology and clinical medicine. Students commenced their medical studies with courses relating to the basic medical sciences and, having completed these, they progressed to clinically-based courses. In recent years, this sequence of courses in the curriculum has been questioned. Early clinical experience has been shown to have major advantages. By demonstrating relevance it motivates students and leads to more effective learning of the basic sciences. It orientates the medical curriculum towards the social context of medicine and eases students' transition to the clinical environment. It also influences students' career choice.

There is a strong argument for continuing the study of the basic medical sciences into the later years of the course. Peter Garland, former professor of biochemistry at the University of Dundee, proposed that the biochemistry course be scheduled in the later years of the curriculum rather than in the early years. He was of the view that students would as a result be better equipped to appreciate the importance of the biochemistry they were studying.

PROGRESSION

The sequence of courses in the curriculum should enable students to progress continuously towards the exit learning outcomes, with the learning outcomes at each stage being challenging and achievable.

Four dimensions can be considered in relation to students' progression through the curriculum (Harden 2007):

1. *Increased breadth.* As they progress through the programme, the learners can extend their area of competence to new topics and to different practice contexts. In clinical medicine, for example, they can learn about heart murmurs not previously considered and learn about an aspect of medicine as applied to children as distinct from adults.
2. *Increased difficulty.* Students can progress by gaining a greater understanding through addressing a learning outcome in more depth. They may learn more about the pathogenesis of a disease or be able to interpret an atypical example of a cardiac murmur already studied.
3. *Increased utility and application to practice.* Students can progress from a more theoretical understanding of a subject to its application in medical practice. In the early years students may practise communication skills with their colleagues or with simulated patients. In the later years they move on to communicate with patients in a range of clinical settings, at first supervised and later unsupervised.
4. *Increased proficiency.* Students may demonstrate increased proficiency in an area associated with more efficient and effective performance. This may be exemplified by less time required for a clinical task or the achievement of higher standards with fewer errors.

The four dimensions are described in Appendix 10.

A SPIRAL CURRICULUM

Relevant to the concept of sequencing is the idea of a spiral curriculum where there is an iterative revisiting of topics, subjects or themes. A spiral curriculum is not simply the repetition of the topic taught. It requires the deepening of understanding with each successive encounter building on the previous one. The following are the features of a spiral curriculum:

- **Topics are revisited.** Students revisit topics, themes or subjects on a number of occasions during a course. A body system such as the cardiovascular system may be studied in the early years and again at a later stage in the curriculum.
- **There are increasing levels of difficulty.** The topics visited are addressed in successive levels of difficulty. Each return visit has added learning outcomes and presents fresh learning opportunities to help the student work towards the final learning outcomes.
- **New learning is related to previous learning.** New information or skills introduced are related back and linked directly to learning in previous phases of the spiral. For example a cardiovascular system course in year 3 of a curriculum will build on the understanding of normal structure and function achieved in the cardiovascular course in year 1. In a third loop in the

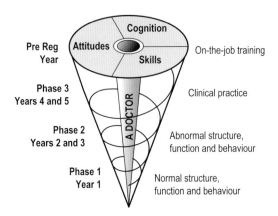

FIG 12.1 An example of a spiral curriculum. (Modified from Harden and Stamper, 1999.)

spiral in the final year, students have the opportunity to study cardiovascular problems in the context of patients they see in their clinical attachments.

- **Competence of students increases.** The learner's competence increases with each visit until the final learning outcomes are achieved.

TRANSITION BETWEEN COURSES

As students progress through the curriculum it is important that the transition between the different phases or courses is as seamless as possible. To facilitate this, a bridging programme may be necessary. Transition courses may take into account students' individual achievements and competencies and ensure that they have the prerequisites necessary for the next step in their training programme. Should deficiencies be identified, learning opportunities can be provided to fill the gaps. Transition programmes are particularly important at the interface between undergraduate and postgraduate programmes before students take up their first medical appointment as trainee doctors. Such a programme may include a period of shadowing a senior doctor in post or a review of the practical skills expected of a junior doctor with remediation where necessary. Induction programmes can introduce the new doctor to administrative and procedural arrangements and to other members of the team.

REFLECT AND REACT

1. Think of your own course in the context of a spiral curriculum. Does it help students to build on what they already know? What will your course add?
2. If students fail to master the learning outcomes for your course, is there a remediation plan in place to help them before they move on to the next phase of their training?
3. Is there a need for an orientation or transitional course between your own course and what precedes or follows it?

IF YOU HAVE A FEW HOURS

Dornan, T., Littlewood, S., Margolis, S.A., et al., 2006. How can experience in clinical and community settings contribute to early medical education? A BEME systematic review. BEME Guide No. 6. Med. Teach. 28, 13–18.
The rationale for the early introduction of clinical experience in the medical curriculum.

Harden, R.M., 2007. Learning outcomes as a tool to assess progression. Med. Teach. 29, 678–682.

Harden, R.M., Stamper, N., 1999. What is a spiral curriculum? Med. Teach. 21, 141–143.
A description of the concept of a spiral curriculum.

Harden, R.M., Davis, M.H., Crosby, J.R., 1997. The new Dundee medical curriculum: a whole that is greater than the sum of the parts. Med. Educ. 31, 264–271.
A case study of a spiral curriculum in action.

Adopting a student-centred approach

The role of the teacher has to change when we empower students to take more responsibility for their own learning.

THE MOVE FROM TEACHER-CENTRED TO STUDENT-CENTRED LEARNING

The two key inhabitants of the medical school are the students and the teachers, with a major focus on the teacher and what is taught. There has been a significant shift in emphasis from the teacher to the student and what the student learns. In this move from teacher-centred to student-centred learning, the role of the teacher has changed from one of information provider to a facilitator of learning – from being a 'sage on the stage' to a 'guide on the side' (Figure 13.1). This concept of student-centred learning underpins much of what this book is about.

A teacher-centred approach emphasises prescribed learning experiences, courses or programmes with a set range of formal activities. It can be likened to eating in a restaurant with a table d'hôte menu where the diners have to eat what the restaurateur chooses. The student-centred approach in contrast is more like an á la carte menu where the diners choose what they want to eat from the menu of options provided. Teacher-centred and student-centred learning differ with regard to the student's engagement with content, the teaching and learning methods, the responsibility for learning, assessment and the balance of power (Table 13.1).

REASONS FOR THE MOVE

The move to student-centred learning has taken place for a number of reasons:

- Student-centred learning is more motivating for students. As Winston Churchill said, 'Personally, I am always ready to learn, although I do not always like being taught'.
- In today's consumer-driven society there is more interest in the student as a consumer of the learning.
- Students are admitted to study medicine from more diverse backgrounds with varying learning needs.

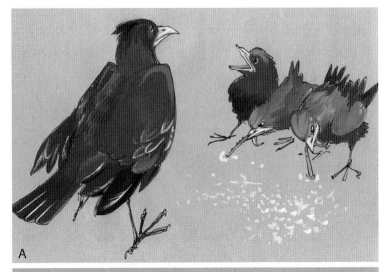

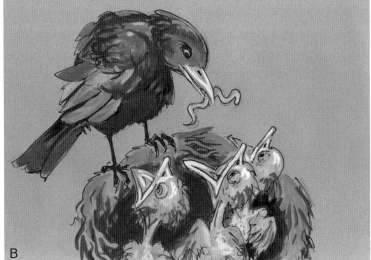

FIG 13.1 The teacher is a facilitator of learning (A) rather than an information provider (B).

- The concept of outcome-based education embraces a commitment to ensure that all students achieve the expected learning outcomes. How they do this will vary from student to student.
- Student-centred learning prepares the student to take responsibility for continuing learning after completion of their undergraduate and postgraduate studies.
- New learning technologies, as described in Section 4, are available which give students more control over their learning.
- Students react positively when allowed to make decisions about their own learning. This is reflected in the extract from a student's diary shown in Box 13.1.

	Teacher-centred	Student-centred
Table 13.1 *A comparison between student-centred and teacher-centred learning (adapted from Blumberg, 2009)*		
Engagement with content	Students learn and memorise content as presented by the teacher	The students reflect on the content and make their own sense out of it
Relation of the teaching and learning methods to the student's learning outcomes	The teacher does not relate the teaching to the learning outcomes	The teacher uses a variety of methods and matches these to the student's achievement of the learning outcomes
Responsibility for learning	The teacher takes responsibility for teaching and assumes that the student will learn	The teacher provides the students with increasing responsibility for their own learning
Assessment	The teacher does not integrate assessment with the learning	Assessment is integrated with the learning process
Balance of power	Decisions about the course, the approaches adopted, the policies and the deadlines are taken by the teacher	The student is engaged with decisions about the curriculum

BOX 13.1 Extracts from the diary of a student studying a course where lectures were replaced with independent learning resource material

At the beginning of the course:
'What, no lectures?'
1 week later:
'I would prefer a lecture course with the optional extra of working on the computer.'
2 weeks later:
'I would now choose a course combining e-learning with printed material and occasional lectures.'
4 weeks later:
'I believe the lecture course should be scrapped. It is a waste of time. I learn better at my own rate on the computer. Now I have time to learn about endocrinology instead of just collecting a set of lecture notes.'

THE ROLE OF THE TEACHER

In student-centred learning the teacher still has an important role to play. The teacher's responsibilities include:

- clarifying expected learning outcomes
- assessing the student's knowledge and skills in relation to the topic
- working with the student to plan the most appropriate sequence and pace of learning
- advising the student about the available learning opportunities to meet their personal needs

- providing formal instruction where this is necessary
- directing the student to tools which they can use to assess their achievement of the learning outcomes
- offering remedial advice where this is required and reassessing the student's achievements.

Student-centred learning does not mean that the teacher abandons the students to their own devices. 'Self-directed learning' has been used to describe the approach. A more appropriate term is 'directed self-learning' as students need some form of help or direction. The extent to which the teacher controls or directs the student or trainee will vary over time. Dron (2007) suggests that 'the optimal degree of learner control at any point will exist somewhere between the two extremes, complete autonomy and total control by another. The difficult task for both teacher and learner is to decide exactly where that point is. A perfect educational system would be one that offers the learner the means to choose at any point what level of control he or she may exercise'.

THE USE OF STUDY GUIDES

A question to be asked is 'How can the teacher support the students' learning, particularly when there may be limitations on how much on-going support or time the teacher has available to devote to individual students or trainees?'. One answer is for the teacher to provide the student with a study guide. Rowntree (1990) has equated a study guide to a tutor sitting on the student's shoulders, available 24 hours a day as required. The guide can be print-based or made available electronically. The purpose is to facilitate learning by describing how the student can best interact with the range of learning opportunities available in order to meet the expected learning outcomes.

Study guides outline the specific learning outcomes to be achieved of the student, specify the range of available learning resources with information on how the resources can be accessed, and provide information about assessment.

A study guide has three elements:

1. *A management function.* Students are offered advice about what they should be learning – the learning outcomes – and the range of learning opportunities available. As they work through the learning programme they are guided on how they can assess their progress, how they can make best use of their time, and what they can do if they encounter difficulties. The study guide can offer encouragement to the learner.
2. *A set of activities.* Activities embedded in the guide can require a student to apply their newly acquired knowledge and skills in practice whether it is with a simulated patient scenario or in a real clinical context. The student can be advised, for example, of the types and numbers of patients they should see in the clinical setting and the procedures they should carry out.

3. *Content.* A study guide should not be confused with or replace a textbook. It may contain information about the topic not readily available from another source. It can put what the student is learning in a local context and can provide updated content where there have been recent changes in practice.

The level of sophistication or complexity of a study guide will vary. Sophisticated study guides have been produced as part of major projects or as part of a curriculum development activity. Less complex study guides can be produced more quickly by teachers for their own course, yet still be of value to the students. The template provided in Appendix 2 will help with the design of a guide. A page from a study guide is given in Appendix 4.

ADAPTIVE LEARNING

A development of student-centred learning is the concept of adaptive learning. An adaptive curriculum recognises that the student body is not a homogenous group and that students differ in their preferred learning styles, interests and abilities. The provision of a range of learning opportunities allows students, with advice from the teacher or trainer, to select those that best suit their personal needs.

Traditionally, the time allocated for a student to complete a course or curriculum is fixed. What varies is the standard students reach. In a truly student-centred approach what is constant is the standard reached, with the variable being the time taken for the student to reach the standard. In this way the course accommodates the slow and the fast learner.

It could be argued that medical schools and postgraduate training programmes have become too rigid with too little freedom for the student or trainee to follow their own interests and select a learning strategy appropriate to their own needs. With the use of new technologies and e-learning, an almost infinite range of experiences can be provided for students to address their individual needs. The delivery of adaptive learning is likely to be a significant development in the years ahead.

REFLECT AND REACT

1. Most teachers believe that students should assume responsibility for their own learning, but their behaviour as a teacher does not support this philosophy. Where does your own approach lie on the continuum between student-centred and teacher-centred approaches?
2. Think what you might be able to do in your situation to make your programme more student-centred, for example in the dimensions noted in Figure 13.1.
3. If your course lacks a study guide why not prepare one yourself? Your students will greatly appreciate your efforts.
4. The implementation of a fully adaptive curriculum is unlikely to be possible at present. Think about the actions you might take to align the teaching and learning programme more closely to the individual needs of each student or trainee.

EXPLORING FURTHER

IF YOU HAVE A FEW HOURS

Harden, R.M., 2009. Independent learning. In: Dent, J.A., Harden, R.M. (Eds.), A Practical Guide for Medical Teachers. third ed. Elsevier, London, pp. 168–173 (Chapter 21).
The six key principles of independent learning are outlined in this chapter.

Harden, R.M., Laidlaw, J.M., Hesketh, E.A., 1999. Study guides – their use and preparation. AMEE Medical Education Guide No. 16 Med. Teach. 21, 248–265.

IF YOU HAVE MORE TIME

Blumberg, P., 2009. Developing Learner-Centred Teaching. A Practical Guide for Faculty. Jossey-Bass, San Francisco.

Dron, J., 2007. Control and Constraint in E-Learning, Choosing when to Choose. Idea Group Publishing, London.
A useful account of when students should be given autonomy on their learning.

Rowntree, D., 1990. Teaching Through Self-Instruction. Kogan Page Ltd, London.
This book will be of help to you if you are planning to develop self-instruction material. It also provides practical advice on teaching with self-instruction.

Building learning around problems and clinical presentations

A clinical problem or task undertaken by a healthcare professional can serve as the basis for learning. The student is motivated by the more authentic learning experience.

A traditional medical course focused on imparting to students the large body of basic science and clinical knowledge and the skills required of a doctor. An alternative focus for students' learning is the problems, clinical presentations or tasks undertaken by a doctor.

PROBLEM-BASED-LEARNING (PBL)

DEFINITION

Problem-based learning has been widely adopted in medical education as an education strategy but its use has not been without controversy. The principal idea behind PBL is that the starting point for the learning is a clinical problem. This is the focus for the student's learning and drives the learning activities on a 'need to know' basis. PBL has made a major contribution to medical education, but there has been a lack of clarity or a conceptual fog surrounding what is meant by the term. The underpinning educational principle is that students, when presented with examples from clinical practice, work out the principles or rules from the basic and clinical sciences that allow them to understand and interpret the problem (Fig. 15.1).

REASONS FOR A MOVE TO PBL

PBL offers a number of advantages, if implemented correctly:

- Students find the process enjoyable and motivating.
- Students are actively engaged in the learning. Activity is one of the FAIR principles for effective learning described in Chapter 2.
- Learning is related to medical practice and is seen by students as relevant – another FAIR principle.
- PBL addresses learning outcomes such as teamwork and problem solving, competencies often overlooked in the conventional curriculum.
- PBL encourages the development of an integrated body of knowledge that is usable in future clinical practice.

IMPLEMENTATION OF PBL

Approaches have varied as to the steps in the process, the nature and format of 'the problem', and the level of support given to students. PBL is based usually on small group work, with 8–10 students per group, although larger numbers of students can be engaged. A member of staff usually facilitates the group, but students can act as facilitators. Although small group work is seen by some as an essential feature of PBL, the technique can be used in the lecture situation or with individual students working independently online.

An example of the steps in the PBL process is described below. The sequence is normally completed over the course of a week.

1. Students receive the problem scenario. Traditionally this has been in print format, typically a short description of a patient's presentation. The problem may be presented using a multi-media approach with a computer, video-tape or simulator. Simulated patients have also been used.
2. Students identify and clarify unfamiliar terms, then define and agree the problem or problems to be discussed. It is important that students do not spend too much time figuring out what they should learn at the expense of time spent learning.
3. Students consider possible explanations of the situation presented on the basis of their prior knowledge and identify areas where further learning is required. The tutor helps to ensure that the learning outcomes identified by the student are appropriate taking into account the learning outcomes for the course and what is achievable in the time available.
4. Students work independently and gather information relating to the learning outcomes. The group may agree to subdivide the task and allocate different responsibilities to individual members. Some of this work may be done online in the small group setting using a search engine such as Google.
5. The group reconvenes and shares the results of their private study. What they learn is then applied to the problem presented.
6. Additional information about the patient may be presented to the students and the above process is repeated.

Various points have been defined on the continuum between a problem-based approach and an information-orientated approach as described in the SPICES model (Harden and Davis 1999). This is summarised in Appendix 9. PBL is usually adopted in the context of an integrated medical curriculum but the strategy can also be used in a curriculum where the emphasis is on subjects or disciplines.

Much of the work with PBL has taken place in the context of the early years of undergraduate education but the strategy has a role to play in the later years of undergraduate education and in postgraduate and continuing education. In continuing education the doctor may work individually at a distance with problems presented online or paper-based.

THE ROLE OF THE TEACHER

There has been much study and debate about the role of the teacher in PBL. His or her role can include:

- **Facilitating the learning in the small group.** There is general agreement that the tutor must have skills in facilitation. The tutor need not be a subject expert in the area but some medical knowledge is helpful (although not everyone agrees with this). The greatest problem to arise in the delivery of PBL relates to the quality of the input from the teachers and their ability to act as facilitators in the PBL setting. PBL sessions should not degenerate into a tutorial dominated by the tutor. Staff training to prevent this happening is important.
- **Assessment of the student.** The teacher may be responsible for assessing and recording the performance of the PBL group and the individual student's performance in the group. This may relate both to their mastery of the subject and to their performance and their skills as a group member. Student assessment is discussed in Section 5.
- **Provision of resource materials.** An area of controversy is the extent to which resource materials relating to the subject should be made available to students. Some teachers favour supporting students' learning by providing extensive handouts and background information that covers the key areas to be studied. Others believe that students should not be 'spoon fed' and that it should be left to the student to identify and locate relevant material. If students are to achieve the expected learning outcomes within the set timescale, it is important that they are not faced with unnecessary difficulties or barriers.
- **Presentation of the problem.** The teacher may also have an input to the development of the problem and to its presentation in print or multi-media format.
- **Curriculum planning.** The contribution of PBL to the course learning outcomes needs to be made explicit. PBL small group work needs to be integrated with other elements within the curriculum. Lectures may still have a useful part to play as well as clinical and other practical work.

TASK-BASED LEARNING

DEFINITION

Task-based learning (TBL) incorporates the same educational philosophy as PBL and indeed has been described as part of the PBL continuum as illustrated in Appendix 9 (Harden and Davis 1999). In task-based learning the focus for the learner is not a paper problem simulation but the description of a task addressed by healthcare professionals. An example is 'the management of a patient with abdominal pain'. In task-based learning the objective is not simply to learn to perform the task but to learn about the basic and clinical sciences relevant to the task and in so doing to gain a more in-depth understanding of the task (Figure 14.1). TBL recognises the need to know not only how to do

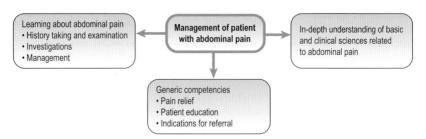

FIG 14.1 In TBL learning occurs round a task.

something but also the principles or basis underlying the required action. In the abdominal pain example, the student's attention is focused on issues such as the relevant anatomy and physiology of the abdomen, on the understanding of the mechanism of pain, on abdominal pathologies, and on the different approaches to investigation and management of a patient with abdominal pain.

TBL IN A CLINICAL SETTING

TBL is useful as an approach to curriculum integration and PBL in the clinical clerkships (Harden et al 2000). In the example given of the management of a patient with abdominal pain, students may concentrate on different aspects of the task in each of the clerkships through which they rotate:

- Acute abdominal pain and the emergency diagnosis and management in a surgical clerkship.
- Approaches to the investigation of a patient in a medical clerkship.
- Specific aspects relating to gynaecological causes in a gynaecological clerkship.
- Age-related differences in a geriatric or paediatric attachment.
- Psychosomatic aspects in a psychiatry attachment.
- The roles of different members of the healthcare team, early diagnosis, decision making and coping with uncertainty in a General Practice attachment. When for example should a patient complaining of abdominal pain be investigated and referred to hospital?
- Geographical and cultural differences in an overseas elective.

TBL places more responsibility on the student and serves to integrate learning across the range of clinical rotations in an undergraduate curriculum or postgraduate training programme.

IMPLEMENTATION OF TBL

Medical schools that adopt a TBL approach generate usually about 100–150 clinical presentations as the focus for the curriculum. A list of the 104 presentations adopted in one school is given in Appendix 3. Grids or blueprints should be produced that identify how each task contributes to the learning outcomes and to the range of learning experiences in which the students engage. As described above, abdominal pain is a focus for the students' learning in a range of clinical clerkships, each contributing in a different way to the students' mastery of the learning outcomes of the course.

TBL provides a structure and focus for postgraduate education that previously was all too often lacking. It helps resolve what may be perceived to be a conflict between service delivery and the education of the student or trainee. Six tasks performed routinely by trainee dentists were identified as the basis for a postgraduate dental training programme. The expected learning outcomes were specified for each task as illustrated in the grid in Appendix 11.

The tasks specified in the curriculum documents can provide a framework for a student's portfolio and this can be used for assessment as described in Chapter 31.

REFLECT AND REACT

1. PBL has proved attractive as an educational strategy for many teachers who have been intent on improving their courses. Others have been reluctant to adopt a teaching approach that seems alien to what they believe to be 'good teaching'. Where do you stand? If you are a sceptic you may be converted if you see examples of good PBL in practice and talk with the students and other teachers who are involved.
2. Where are you on the PBL continuum as described in Appendix 9?
3. If you have adopted PBL in your teaching do you make full use of the new technologies to present the problem to the learner?
4. If you have undergraduate or postgraduate responsibilities for clinical teaching, you may wish to explore the concept of TBL. It may also be used to introduce a clinical focus in the early years of the curriculum.

EXPLORING FURTHER

IF YOU HAVE A FEW HOURS

Colliver, J.A., 2000. Effectiveness of problem-based learning curricula: research and theory. Acad. Med. 75, 259–266.
A review of problem-based learning.

Davis, M.H., Harden, R.M., 1999. Problem-based Learning: A Practical Guide. AMEE Medical Education Guide No. 15 AMEE, Dundee.
The underpinning principles and an outline of the advantages and disadvantages of the approach.

Harden, R.M., Davis, M.H., 1999. The continuum of problem-based learning. Med. Teach. 20, 317–322.
A model for analysing the level at which PBL is introduced into a curriculum.

Harden, R.M., Crosby, J.R., Davis, M.H., et al., 2000. Task-based learning: the answer to integration and problem-based learning in the clinical years. Med. Educ. 34, 391–397.
A description of TBL in the clinical years of a medical school's programme.

Harden, R.M., Laidlaw, J.M., Ker, J.S., Mitchell, H.E., 1998. Task Based Learning: An educational Strategy for Undergraduate, Postgraduate and Continuing Medical Education. AMEE Medical Education Guide No. 7 AMEE, Dundee.
An introduction to TBL. Eight aspects of implementing TBL are described in this Guide.

Taylor, D., Miflin, B., 2010. Problem-Based Learning: Where Are We Now? AMEE Medical Education Guide No. 36 AMEE, Dundee.
A current review of the role of problem-based learning in medicine.

IF YOU HAVE MORE TIME

Barrows, H.S., Tamblyn, R.M., 1980. Problem-Based Learning: An Approach to Medical Education. Springer Publishing Company, New York.

Schwartz, P., Mennin, S., Webb, G. (Eds.), Problem-Based Learning. Kogan Page Ltd, London.
A description of problem-based learning in action.

Using an integrated and inter-professional approach

An integrated curriculum, bringing together different disciplines, offers major advantages. There are also benefits from sharing learning experiences with different professions.

DEFINITION

The most significant change that has taken place globally in medical education since the 1970s has been the move from curricula that focused on individual subjects or disciplines to a programme where the teaching and learning are integrated. In a traditional discipline-based curriculum, subjects were taught in separate courses, each with its own programme of lectures and its own assessment. Students learned about the structure of the heart in the anatomy course at a different time from learning about the function of the heart in the physiology course, the cardiac drugs in the pharmacology course and abnormalities of the heart in the pathology course. With an integrated approach the different subjects are brought together, most typically around a body system such as the cardiovascular system.

The term 'horizontal integration' is used to describe the bringing together of subjects in the same phase of the curriculum. 'Vertical integration' is applied to the integration of subjects normally taught in different phases of the curriculum. Traditionally, the early years of the medical course were devoted to the study of the basic medical sciences. More recently we have seen, as described in Chapter 11, the introduction of clinical learning opportunities into the earlier years and the basic sciences related to this. More attention needs to be

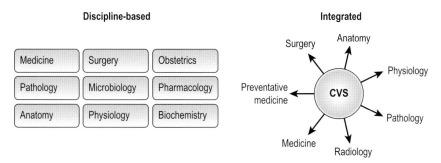

FIG 15.1 A comparison between how subjects are covered in a discipline-based and integrated curriculum.

paid to the integration of the basic sciences with clinical medicine in the later years of the curriculum.

ADVANTAGES OF INTEGRATION

Having emerged from the shadows as an alternative approach to curriculum development, integration has become the standard approach to curriculum development in many medical schools worldwide. There are a number of reasons for this:

- **Integrated teaching reflects the practice of medicine.** An integrated approach, more than a discipline-based approach, encourages the student to take a holistic view of the patient and his or her problems. In a final examination in a medical school that had a discipline-based curriculum we observed that a student, when asked to take a history from a woman with abdominal pain, enquired whether he should take a medical, surgical or gynaecological history. He had clearly failed to integrate what he had learned in the different clinical attachments.
- **Integration motivates the students.** Most students are not interested in becoming anatomists or physiologists and the relevance of the basic sciences to the practice of medicine may not be appreciated by them. The traditional curriculum, sadly, was often associated with a decrease in the early years in the students' enthusiasm and interest in medicine.
- **Integration by relating theory to practice makes learning more effective.** The ability to retrieve an item from memory depends on the similarity between the condition in which it was learned and the context in which it is to be retrieved. In the classic diver experiment, divers learned from a text underwater and on the surface. When tested subsequently on the surface they performed better on the text learned on the surface. When tested underwater they performed better on the text they had learned underwater. This has been replicated in many other studies. It is also recognised that knowledge learned in isolation and not applied is easily forgotten – so called 'inert' knowledge.
- **An integrated curriculum can help to avoid unnecessary re-duplication.** An integrated curriculum highlights what is important for the student to know and can be seen as a response to the problem of information overload.
- **The integrated curriculum may be more cost effective.** Greater efficiency can be achieved by sharing teaching and learning resources such as the facilities in a clinical skills laboratory.
- **An integrated approach promotes collaboration and communication between staff.** An integrated approach requires a discussion between staff as to how each subject can contribute to the learning outcomes. Staff who collaborate in their teaching may go on to collaborate in their research activities.

FOCUS FOR INTEGRATION

The focus for integration may be:

- **The body systems.** This is the most commonly adopted approach in the early years of the medical course with students studying, for example, a 6-week course on the cardiovascular system, a 5-week course on the respiratory system, etc.

- **The life cycle.** A focus for the integration may be the life cycle including the newborn, the child, the adolescent, the adult, the elderly and death. This may be used in conjunction with a system-based approach.
- **Clinical presentations or a set of descriptions of the tasks facing a doctor.** Task-based learning as described in Chapter 14 and in Appendix 3 is a useful approach to integration, particularly in the later years of the course (Harden et al 2000).

THE INTEGRATION CONTINUUM

Discussions about integration have been polarised with some teachers arguing in favour and others against integrated teaching. In the SPICES model for educational strategies, integration is presented as a continuum with full integration at one end and discipline-based teaching at the other (Harden 2000). Any position between the two extremes may be adopted as described on the integration ladder (Fig. 15.2). The most appropriate level to suit a particular curriculum can be identified.

Step 1 – Isolation

Departments or subject specialists, represented by squares in the diagram, organise their teaching in isolation with no consideration of other subjects or disciplines.

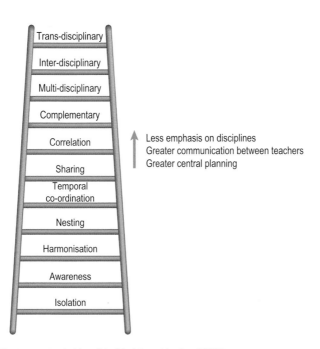

FIG 15.2 The integration ladder. (Modified from Harden, 2000.)

Using an integrated and inter-professional approach

Step 2 – Awareness

The teaching is subject-based as in Step 1 but some mechanisms are in place whereby a teacher in one subject is made aware of what is covered in other subjects in the curriculum.

Step 3 – Harmonisation

In harmonisation, teachers responsible for different courses consult each other and communicate about their courses.

Step 4 – Nesting

In this integrated approach the teacher includes, within a subject-based course, knowledge and skills relating to other subjects.

Step 5 – Temporal co-ordination

The timetable is adjusted so that related topics within subjects are scheduled at the same time, with similar topics being taught on the same day or week.

Step 6 – Sharing

Two disciplines implement the teaching programme and some teaching is shared between the departments.

Step 7 – Correlation

In addition to the subject-based teaching, an integrated teaching session is introduced that brings together areas of common interest in each of the subjects.

Step 8 – Complementary programme

There is both subject-based and integrated teaching but with integrated sessions representing a major feature of the curriculum.

Step 9 – Multi-disciplinary

A number of subjects are brought together in a single course with an integrated theme, but with the subjects clearly identified.

Step 10 – Inter-disciplinary

Subjects lose their identity in a new integrated programme.

Step 11 – Trans-disciplinary

The integration is built around the field of knowledge as exemplified in the real world rather than a theme or topic selected for the purpose.

INTER-PROFESSIONAL EDUCATION

DEFINITION

Integrated teaching as described above is concerned with bringing together the disciplines within medicine. Inter-professional education occurs when two or more different professions learn with, from and about each other. In medical practice today, no one profession can respond adequately to the range of problems presented by patients. It is essential that doctors have the necessary teamwork skills and understanding of different roles if they are to work alongside nurses, pharmacists, physiotherapists, health visitors and other members of the healthcare team. The education of doctors has been largely conducted in the past in a silo with little consideration given to the other professions and almost no collaboration with regard to joint educational programmes. Inter-professional education enables the knowledge and skills necessary for collaborative working to be learned and can result in an improvement in the delivery of healthcare.

CONTINUUM OF INTER-PROFESSIONAL EDUCATION

Inter-professional education can be described along a continuum of 11 stages, from isolation where healthcare professionals are taught separately from each other with no contact, to trans-professional education where learning is based in practice (Harden 1999). The steps are similar to the steps described on the integration ladder.

PRINCIPLES OF INTER-PROFESSIONAL LEARNING

The Centre for the Advancement of Interprofessional Education (CAIPE) in the UK developed seven principles to guide provision, commissioning and development of inter-professional education (Freeth 2010). The vision is that inter-professional education:

1. works to improve the quality of care
2. focuses on the needs of service users and carers
3. involves service users and carers
4. encourages professions to learn with, from and about each other
5. respects the integrity and contribution of each profession
6. enhances practice within the professions
7. increases professional satisfaction.

IMPLEMENTATION

Inter-professional education is generally well received, enabling knowledge and skills necessary for collaborative working to be learned (Hammick et al 2007). Methods used to implement inter-professional education in practice as described by Barr (2009) include:

- exchange-based learning: for example debates, case studies, shared lectures and e-learning

- action-based learning: for example problem-based learning (PBL) and task-based learning (TBL)
- observation-based learning: for example joint visits to a patient by students from different professions, shadowing another professional and work-related practice placements
- simulation-based learning: for example role-play, games, skills lab and a simulated ward
- portfolios and assessment.

Resource materials may be developed that highlight inter-professional practice. We worked with a multi-professional team from Africa to develop a training handbook for use by members of the healthcare team. The handbook was based on the common clinical problems encountered by healthcare professionals in their daily work, e.g. a patient with diarrhoea. A general account of the management of the problem was provided in the top half of each page. In the three columns on the bottom half of the page there was a description of the roles of the doctor, the nurse and the health officer. The team members were able to master the skills relating to their own roles, while gaining an understanding of the roles of other members of the healthcare team.

How inter-professional education is implemented is important and may determine the success of the approach. Multi-professional PBL groups may succeed or fail depending on the nature of the presenting problem, the briefing of the group, the facilitation by the tutor and the debriefing. PBL worked effectively in our experience with a group of trainee midwives and medical students, when the task facing the group required both the practical experience of the trainee midwives and the theoretical understanding of the medical students. The result was a positive shift in attitude of medical students towards midwives and vice versa. Other reported experiences of multi-professional groups have been less successful.

REFLECT AND REACT

1. Think about the approach to integration in your course. What is the focus for the integration and where are you on the integration ladder?
2. If you have an integrated curriculum, do the learning outcomes, the learning opportunities provided and the assessment all reflect an integrated approach?
3. In planning and implementing your training programme, has an inter-professional approach been considered? Have you discussed this with teachers in other professions?

EXPLORING FURTHER

IF YOU HAVE A FEW HOURS

Barr, H., 2009. Interprofessional education. In: Dent, J.A., Harden, R.M. (Eds.), A Practical Guide for Medical Teachers, third ed. Elsevier, London Chapter 24).
A useful account of interprofessional education.

Hammick, M., Freeth, D., Koppel, I., Reeves, S., Barr, H., 2007. The best evidence systematic review of interprofessional education. BEME Guide No. 9 Med. Teach. 29, 735–751.
A description of inter-professional education and the educational principles underpinning successful shared learning.

Hammick, M., Olckers, L., Campion-Smith, C., 2009. Learning in Interprofessional Teams. AMEE Guide No. 38. AMEE, Dundee.
An overview of the place of inter-professional education in the healthcare professions.

Harden, R.M., 1999. Multiprofessional Education. AMEE Medical Education Guide 12. AMEE, Dundee.
A description of approaches to multi-professional education.

Harden, R.M., 2000. The integration ladder: a tool for curriculum planning and evaluation. Med. Educ. 34, 551–557.
A description of the 11 steps in the integration ladder.

Harden, R.M., Crosby, J., Davis, M.H., et al., 2000. Task-based learning: the answer to integration and problem-based learning in the clinical years. Med. Educ. 34, 391–397.
A description of how TBL provides a focus for integration in the clinical years.

IF YOU HAVE MORE TIME

Bandaranayake, R., 2011. The Integrated Medical Curriculum. Radcliffe Publishing, London.
A definitive and practical account of integration in the medical curriculum.

Fogarty, R., 1991. How to Integrate the Curricula. IRI/Skylight Training and Publishing, Illinois.
A view of the integrated curriculum from the perspective of schools.

Freeth, D., 2010. Interprofessional education. In: Swanwick, T. (Ed.), Understanding Medical Education: Evidence, Theory and Practice. Wiley-Blackwell, Chichester (Chapter 4).

Miller, B.M., Moore Jr., D.E., Stead, W.W., et al., 2010. Beyond Flexner: a new model for continuous learning in the health professions. Acad. Med. 85, 266–272.
This article describes a model that promotes inter-professional education.

Using an integrated and inter-professional approach

Making the apprenticeship model and work-based learning more effective

There is no better way to learn than from work-related experience. This requires careful monitoring and supervision.

THE APPRENTICESHIP

In the nineteenth century and earlier, doctors were trained as apprentices to practising doctors. The master accepted the pupil, who paid for the privilege and was taught and instructed in the methods and secrets (Calman 2006). In the late nineteenth and early part of the twentieth century the lack of attention to the scientific basis of medicine in undergraduate education and the varying quality of the apprenticeship experience offered led to a significant shift towards a university-based education. The emphasis was placed on more formal and theoretical education in the classroom and on the didactic lecture.

Over the years growing disquiet has been expressed about the removal of much of the education from the clinical setting and today greater emphasis is again being placed on learning on the job. The learning experience, however, is being more carefully arranged and monitored; on-the-job learning is now incorporated and plays a key role as part of a more formal planned curriculum.

DEFINITION

Work-based learning (WBL) is a key strategy in postgraduate and continuing education but it is relevant too in undergraduate education. It can be seen as a continuum that stretches from formalised training at one end where a student or junior doctor learns under supervision through to an established practitioner sharing a clinical problem with colleagues.

A number of terms have been used to describe work-based learning (WBL). These include on-the-job learning (OJL), service-based learning, experience-based learning, learning from practice, situated learning and community-based learning. The key feature is that students or trainees participate in authentic activities that form the basis for their learning. They learn from their experience and at the same time are helped to generalise from the patient they have seen to other patients and situations. Students or trainees learn 'on the job' while 'doing the job'. Learning in the workplace enables students to learn about the context in which they will later practise.

PRINCIPLES

WBL has powerful learning potential. A key underlying principle is that learning is inherent in everyday practice. The core condition for WBL is 'supported participation'. This involves the learners:

- **taking responsibility** for seeking out and engaging in learning experiences
- **being actively involved** in the context of the task being undertaken in the work situation
- **reflecting** on their learning experiences with mentors, supervisors, teachers and peers
- **interacting** with colleagues and other members of the healthcare team
- **receiving on-going feedback** from mentors, supervisors, teachers and peers.

ADVANTAGES

Learning on the job in the clinical environment offers a number of advantages:

- WBL focuses on real problems in the context of professional practice. Relevance, a key principle for effective learning as described in the FAIR model in Chapter 2, is a feature. It provides students/trainees with the satisfaction of doing a 'real job' in an authentic work setting rather than engaging in an academic exercise.
- WBL requires active participation and feedback – two other elements in the FAIR model. In WBL students learn more effectively through doing and through opportunities to practise, particularly when feedback is provided.
- WBL by its very nature can be designed to meet the needs of the learner – individualisation is the fourth component of the FAIR model.
- WBL offers a multi-professional experience that can help students and trainees to work as a member of a team and develop their professional identity.
- Experience on the job can help students and trainees to make a career choice.
- Students' on-the-job experience, such as shadowing house officers in their final year as medical students, may prepare them for their subsequent posting after qualification. It helps them to become familiar with the work environment in the context of healthcare delivery. It may also help to enhance employment prospects for a particular post.

IMPLEMENTATION

Unfortunately the full potential of WBL is often not realised, and the expected learning outcomes are not achieved. The teacher can take several steps to optimise the potential of WBL in undergraduate education and postgraduate training:

- Plan the experience carefully, matching the learning experiences to the expected learning outcomes. What conditions are the student or trainee expected to see and what procedures are they expected to carry out? Unless planned carefully the school of experience is no school at all.
- Make the expectations explicit and draw up and agree a learning plan with the students/trainees.

- Monitor the learners' progress and provide constructive and timely feedback.
- Recognise the potential contributions of other members of the healthcare team to the students' and trainees' on-the-job experiences. The development of satisfactory relationships is an essential part of the exercise.
- Recognise the importance of the education environment. Students or trainees who are made to feel welcome are more likely to engage actively in the full range of learning opportunities provided and are more likely to play an active role within the team (Fig. 16.1). The concept of the education environment is explored in Chapter 18.
- Make medical students an integral part of the patient's care. This may involve the student participating in ward rounds and in some aspects of the patient's management. A student's notes for example may become part of a patient's records, although this and other students' participation can present a legal challenge.
- The learner may benefit from a job aid that provides step-by-step guidelines on the task expected of them. This is particularly important when the task is lengthy or complex, and when the consequence of error is high. The job aid may be presented in print format or electronically through a mobile device.
- A study guide can help the student or trainee to understand what is expected of them in the work place and how they can obtain the maximum educational benefit from their experiences. The guide will help to relate these experiences to the other elements of the training programme and to relate theory to practice. Additional learning experiences such as the use of simulators that may enrich their experiences in the clinical setting are identified. The use of study guides is described in Chapter 13.

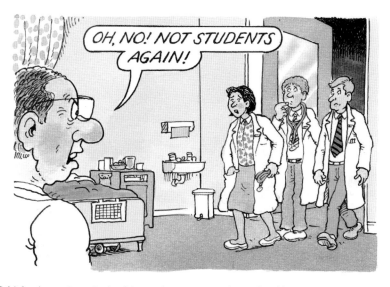

FIG 16.1 A negative attitude of the teacher can impact the students' learning.

Making the apprenticeship model and work-based learning more effective

PROBLEMS AND PITFALLS

Problems and difficulties may be encountered when WBL is implemented:

- The learning may be opportunistic and based solely on the patients seen by the student or trainee. Some repetition of experiences is useful but unnecessary repetition should be avoided. Otherwise the learner is in danger of becoming like the golfer who continues to practise his or her mistakes but does not improve their game.
- The level of responsibility allocated to students or trainees in the delivery of the health care to the patients may present a problem. It is important that learners are not given tasks beyond their capabilities or authority.
- A conflict is sometimes perceived between the educational needs of the doctor in training and the service delivery demands. In WBL the relationship between the education and service components should be made explicit and the education integrated with the service delivery.
- The learners' progress needs to be carefully monitored and appropriate feedback provided. Inappropriate or lack of feedback is a common criticism in WBL (Fig. 16.2). The assessment of the students' progress and their achievement of the learning outcomes can be challenging. Non-traditional methods of assessment may be required and these are discussed in Chapter 31.
- There may be funding implications for the medical school in undergraduate education where money follows the student and in postgraduate training for the hospital where the employment of junior staff may attract high insurance premiums.

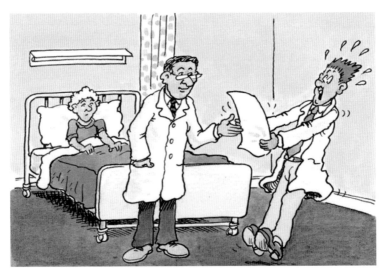

FIG 16.2 Inappropriate feedback may be a problem.

REFLECT AND REACT

1. The work environment has powerful learning potential and can meet the criteria for effective and efficient learning. Is this potential fully achieved with your trainees?
2. As a teacher or trainer think about how you can facilitate and guide learning on the job and provide feedback to the trainee or student.
3. Is there a study guide available to support the student's or trainee's learning? If not, consider preparing one. Extracts from a study guide prepared to support junior doctors during their paediatric training are given in Appendix 4.

EXPLORING FURTHER

IF YOU HAVE A FEW HOURS

Laidlaw, J.M., Harden, R.M., Robertson, L.J., et al., 2003. The design of distance-learning programmes and the role of content experts in their production. Med. Teach. 25, 182–187.
The preparation of a study guide for trainee surgeons is described.

Mitchell, H.E., Harden, R.M., Laidlaw, J.M., 1998. Towards effective on-the-job learning: the development of a paediatric training guide. Med. Teach. 20, 91–98.
A description of how WBL was implemented for junior doctors in a postgraduate paediatric training programme aided by a study guide.

Swanwick, T., 2005. Informal learning in postgraduate medical education: from cognitivism to 'culturism'. Med. Educ. 39, 859–865.
A useful account of work-based learning in practice.

IF YOU HAVE MORE TIME

Calman, K., 2006. Medical Education: Past, Present and Future. Churchill Livingstone, London.
An interesting account of the history of medical education.

Hargreaves, D.H., Bowditch, M.G., Griffin, D.R., 1997a. On-The-Job Training for Surgeons. Royal Society of Medicine Press, London.
A description of the process required for successful on-the-job training for surgeons. While the context of training has changed somewhat since the book was written the key educational messages remain relevant.

Hargreaves, D.H., Southworth, G.W., Stanley, P., Ward, S.J., 1997b. On-The-Job Training for Physicians. Royal Society of Medicine Press, London.
In this book the emphasis is on the training of physicians.

Building options into a core curriculum

Alongside a core curriculum that provides the necessary breadth of study, options and electives provide an opportunity for students to study selected topics in more depth.

BACKGROUND

Information overload is one of the biggest problems facing students today.

Advances in medicine and the so-called 'information explosion' have led to an increasing and potentially intolerable burden for the student. Curriculum committees are expected to pay attention to new topics and topics of particular concern such as team skills, professionalism, pain management, care of the dying, health education and personalised medicine. It has to be recognised, however, that the time available in a curriculum is finite and steps need to be taken to ensure that this time is put to best use.

In responding to the problem of information overload the teacher should:

- Recognise the need for students to move from simple fact memorisation to higher level learning objectives including searching, analysis and

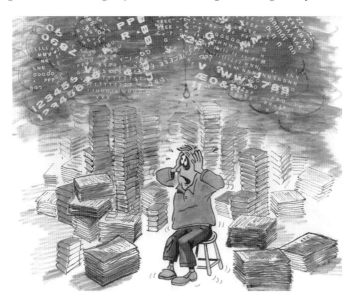

FIG 17.1 Information overload – a major problem facing medical education.

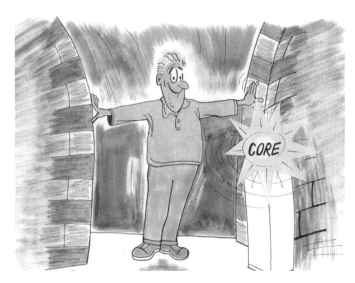

FIG 17.2 Core learning outcomes should be highlighted.

synthesis of information. A theme running throughout the book is the changing role of the teacher from information provider to someone who opens the door for students and allows them to access and retrieve information for themselves.

- Rather than teach more than students are able to learn and expect them to remember only a small proportion when they enter practice, it is preferable in the teaching to emphasise the core or essential learning required.
- Provide the opportunity for students to study in more depth areas of their choosing as either electives or student-selected components (SSCs).

ADVANTAGES OF A CORE CURRICULUM WITH OPTIONS OR STUDENT-SELECTED COMPONENTS (SSCs)

A core curriculum offers a number of advantages:

- It is consistent with outcome-based education and highlights the essential learning requirements for all students.
- It helps to counter the tendency for increasing specialisation in the curriculum.
- It helps to determine the equivalence of training between different programmes and facilitates the mobility of doctors.
- It provides a standard against which students can be assessed.

When combined with options or student-selected components there are additional advantages:

- Students have the opportunity to cover the breadth of knowledge while at the same time they are able to study in depth selected subjects of their choosing.
- Special study modules may be offered in subjects not normally addressed in the curriculum.

- Experience of a subject during an SSC may help students with regard to their career choice. Completion of a series of SSCs in a subject may count towards postgraduate training in that area, shortening the duration of postgraduate training. While unusual at present, this may be more widely recognised in the future.
- Teachers have the benefit of interacting with an enthusiastic group of students who have a special interest in their subject and who might be the researchers or teachers of the future.

SPECIFICATION OF A CORE CURRICULUM

The specification of the core curriculum should be the responsibility of all the stakeholders including the clinicians and basic scientists. It should not be left to each discipline or specialty to specify the core curriculum in their area. The content can be determined as described in Chapter 7.

Topics merit inclusion in a core curriculum if they are:

- common in clinical practice
- representative of a serious or life-threatening situation in clinical practice
- an important prerequisite for other learning and illustrate an important principle.

The core curriculum is reflected in:

- the statement of learning outcomes
- the list of patient presentations that is used as a framework for the curriculum
- the learning opportunities provided for the students, for example experience in the community
- the problems presented in a PBL curriculum
- the assessment.

ELECTIVES/SSCs

A curriculum based on a core with options or electives, as recommended in 1993 by the UK General Medical Council in 'Tomorrow's Doctors', was a major development in curriculum planning. The precise place on the SPICES continuum between a core or uniform curriculum and a curriculum entirely based on student-selected elements requires to be determined by a school. The usual recommendation is that the student-selected component is allocated 10–30% of the available curriculum time.

The concept of electives, often overseas, that provided students with an international focus and the opportunity to experience different cultures is not new. What is different with the 'core and option' curriculum concept is that the options or SSCs are closely integrated into the curriculum and contribute to the core curriculum outcomes. Learning outcomes for the elective curriculum may be content independent and embrace higher order competencies such as independent learning, self-assessment and professionalism. It is through the options that students may have the greatest opportunity to direct their own learning and to assess their own progress.

CHOICE OF SSC TOPICS

A wide range of topics can be addressed in SSCs. These may include:

- A more in-depth study of subjects included in the core curriculum. With a reduction in time allocated to basic sciences in the curriculum, students with an interest in the area have an opportunity to study anatomy or another basic science in more depth.
- Special aspects of clinical practice such as plastic surgery not covered in the curriculum.
- Topics unrelated to medicine but of possible relevance to a doctor's future career, for example the study of a foreign language or business studies.
- Medical education and teaching skills. We have seen students generating useful learning resource material during an SSC.
- Inter-professional experiences, for example working as a member of an inter-professional team or shadowing a nurse. The latter proved a popular SSC in one school but mainly for female students!
- Research: clinical, laboratory-based or educational.

Students may choose from a list of options provided by the medical school or identify their own area for further study.

ASSESSMENT OF SSCs

The assessment of the SSCs should be transparent and related to the contribution the SSC makes to the learning outcomes for the course. The assessment of students' performance in SSCs must be integrated with their overall assessment. Alongside their performance in the core curriculum the SSC assessment should be used to determine their progress.

A range of methods may be used. Portfolio assessment, as described in Chapter 31, offers a number of advantages. Problems relating to fairness and equivalence need to be addressed given the varying nature of different electives.

INTEGRATION OF ELECTIVES WITH THE CORE

SSCs can be integrated in the timetable with the core curriculum in different ways:

- **Sequential.** A block of core teaching, for example 8 weeks, is followed by a 2-week SSC option. This allows the student to explore the subject of the preceding block in more detail, or to study an unrelated subject.
- **Intermittent.** Blocks of time, for example 4–10 weeks, are allocated for SSCs at set times in the curriculum.
- **Concurrent.** The SSC topic is scheduled to run on half or one day per week alongside the core but on a topic not necessarily related to the core.
- **Integrated.** The SSC is integrated within the core topic programme allowing the student to study different aspects of the core in more depth. One option in an endocrinology course we offer is for the student to look at the laboratory investigation of endocrine disease, another to look at surgery and a third to look at the management of endocrine problems in the community.

REFLECT AND REACT

1. Whether you are working in undergraduate or postgraduate training, has the appropriate balance between the core curriculum and SSCs been achieved in your programme?
2. Are the learning outcomes for the SSCs clear to the students and supervisors, and are they assessed appropriately?
3. Is a sufficient choice of SSCs available to students and are they given sufficient guidance to make their choice?

EXPLORING FURTHER

IF YOU HAVE A FEW HOURS

Cholerton, S., Jordan, R., 2009. Core curriculum and student-selected components. In: Dent, J.A., Harden, R.M. (Eds.), A Practical Guide for Medical Teachers. third ed. Elsevier, London, pp. 193–201 (Chapter 25).
A description of how the curriculum with a core and student-selected component should be considered as a whole built round a core set of learning outcomes.

Harden, R.M., Davis, M., 2001. The core curriculum with options or special study modules. AMEE Education Guide No. 5. Med. Teach. 23, 231–244.
A description of the concept and how it can be implemented in practice.

Riley, S.C., 2009. Student selected components. AMEE Guide No. 46. Med. Teach. 31, 885–894.
A guide written for developers of medical curricula where SSC initiatives offer choice and depth of study.

Building options into a core curriculum

Recognising the importance of the education environment

18

This neglected area is now recognised as being a substantial and very real element that influences students' learning. Tools are available to assess the education environment.

WHAT IS THE LEARNING ENVIRONMENT?

We can read the curriculum documents, we can inspect the expected learning outcomes, and we can experience a wide range of teaching approaches, but we may know little about the student's experience in the education programme. Key to this, suggests Genn (2001), is the atmosphere or climate experienced by the student in the school – what is valued, what is recognised and what is encouraged. As Genn describes, the education climate is the soul and heart of the medical school. It is the education environment that determines the students' behaviour, their achievements and their satisfaction. McAleer et al (2009) likened it to the climate or environment in the meteorological context and suggested that we cannot hope to maximise the education output if we do not foster a nurturing climate.

Contributing to the learning environment in a medical school or a postgraduate programme and influencing the students' or trainees' learning, positively or negatively, are:

- how students are taught and the education strategies adopted
- what they are taught
- how they are assessed
- the types of clinical experiences offered
- the books and resources available online or in the library
- the values expressed by their teachers
- physical factors such as lecture theatre seating, heating, cooling and levels of noise.

THE EDUCATION CLIMATE IS IMPORTANT

The establishment of an appropriate climate is almost certainly the most important single task for a medical teacher. Genn and others have highlighted that while the education climate may seem rather intangible, unreal and insubstantial, its effects are pervasive, substantial, very real and influential. The climate, it has been suggested, is like a mist – you cannot stay long in the mist before being thoroughly soaked. The climate includes the type of things

111

© 2012 Elsevier Ltd.

that are rewarded, encouraged and emphasised, and the style of life that is valued in the school or training programme. A study of the learning environment can help to answer questions such as these:

- In the medical school or training programme is collaboration or competition between students encouraged?
- Is the student encouraged to ask questions and think creatively or to participate passively and follow the rules?
- Is the curriculum about meeting the needs of the learner or the needs of the teacher?
- Does the curriculum challenge and stretch students or require only minimum competence?
- Is the environment a trusting one where the teacher is supportive and tolerant of mistakes or is the teacher viewed with suspicion as the 'enemy' of the student?

Without an examination of the education environment these questions go unanswered. Genn (2001) suggests "If we wish to describe, assess, or otherwise 'get a handle on' the curriculum in a medical school, we need to consider the environment, educational and organisational, associated with the curriculum and the medical school".

In postgraduate training particular concerns have related to poor supervision, variable and unpredictable teaching, lack of continuity, the provision of feedback that is not constructive, and an emphasis on service requirements rather than educational requirements. These can all be related to the established education environment.

Suggestions that students become more cynical and less empathetic as they progress through the medical curriculum are a cause of concern. The problem may rest, at least in part, with the education environment. Too often this is task orientated with the emphasis on the presentation by an expert scientist or clinician who knows the answers and procedures while the social–emotional orientation concerning the development of a caring helper of sick people is neglected. An appropriate education environment should encourage the development of abilities to empathise and identify with patients and their predicaments.

The need for a fundamental review of medical education was proposed by the Global Independent Commission on Education of Health Professionals for the 21st Century published in *The Lancet* in December 2010. The recommendations proposed far-reaching changes to learning outcomes and to methods of teaching, learning and assessment and addressed issues relating to teamwork, inter-professional collaboration, international dimensions and individualised learning. One could argue that key to the implementation of these changes is the development of a supportive education environment.

ASPECTS OF THE EDUCATION ENVIRONMENT

The medical education environment is extraordinarily complex. The different dimensions are sometimes referred to as orientations. Some aspects or orientations of the environment that merit consideration are listed here. The list is not comprehensive but it provides examples of the various orientations.

COLLABORATIVE OR COMPETITIVE ORIENTATION

It is a paradox that while teamwork and collaboration are identified as important learning outcomes in medical training and the importance of the inter-professional team is recognised, the training programme with which our students and trainees engage fosters competition rather than collaboration. Students are recognised and rewarded on the basis of their individual performance and not on their performance as a member of a team or group.

A collaborative education environment is created and students develop a feeling of 'belonging' in the group or team if they are encouraged to work with their colleagues and to participate as part of a ward team in clinical attachments. In PBL curricula there have been attempts to value and assess group performance.

STUDENT OR TEACHER ORIENTATION

The education environment may be one in which the teacher is more valued than the student. In a student-centred environment what is valued is the learner, and their interests and student independence and autonomy are encouraged, as discussed in Chapter 13.

SUPPORTIVE OR PUNITIVE ORIENTATION

Students or trainees in the past have been left to their own devices to deal with academic or personal problems. Some students have found the teaching threatening or intimidating, especially if they have been humiliated or harassed. Such an environment has been seen as helping to toughen the student with survival seen as some sort of rite of passage. Learners were encouraged to cover up any difficulties experienced or refrain from divulging gaps in their knowledge. More recently the climate has changed. Students are encouraged to assess their own progress and identify any difficulties they might have with the assurance that support and counselling are available. In a supportive education environment learners are free to experiment, voice their concerns, identify their lack of knowledge and stretch their limits.

COMMUNITY OR HOSPITAL ORIENTATION

Medical education has been criticised as having as its base an ivory tower academic centre, distant from the realities of the day-to-day practice of family medicine in the community. Professors and specialists with international recognition are the role models for the students. It is perhaps not surprising that, in the past, a career in general practice or in a rural community was frowned on by students as being a 'second best' choice. Fortunately this tension has now been recognised and there is a greater emphasis on students learning in the community and in the rural setting with some medical schools established in a rural location.

RESEARCH OR TEACHING ORIENTATION

The teaching and learning programme may be one that is conducted in the context of an environment where research is valued and rewarded, and where teaching is seen as an activity that encroaches on writing research papers or proposals for funding. Some medical schools are trying to redress the balance by recognising the scholarship of teaching as a criterion for appointments and promotions. Newly appointed faculty members may be expected to demonstrate or acquire, through a staff development programme, expertise in teaching.

THE EFFECTS OF THE ENVIRONMENT

The educational climate may manifest itself in a number of ways:

- The education environment makes a unique and notable contribution to the prediction of student achievement and success.
- The motivation of the learner is influenced by the education environment in which he or she is studying.
- Many factors influence career choice but undoubtedly the education environment can have a significant impact. Preference for a career as a surgeon in an academic centre, or for a career as a general practitioner in a rural community, may be attributed to the education environment in the training programme.
- Staff may be more inclined to stay in a post if an institution has a good education environment. It is easier to attract new staff to such an institution.

ASSESSMENT OF THE EDUCATION ENVIRONMENT

One reason why the education environment was ignored in the past was the lack of a suitable instrument or tool to measure it. A number of validated instruments are now available for use in different settings. McAleer et al (2010) described 30 such tools and provided a useful summary of tools available. Those most frequently used are the Dundee Ready Education Environment Measure (DREEM) and the Postgraduate Hospital Educational Environment Measure (PHEEM).

The education environment can be assessed using qualitative as well as quantitative approaches. A qualitative approach involves collecting data using a survey instrument with open-ended questions such as 'What do you most like about your training programme?', or by eliciting feedback from focus groups. With quantitative instruments students are asked to reply to a series of questions with each question relating to one aspect or dimension of the education environment.

DREEM has five subscales as described in Appendix 12:

1. students' perceptions of learning
2. students' perceptions of teachers
3. students' academic self-perceptions
4. students' perceptions of atmosphere
5. students' social self-perceptions.

DREEM contains 50 statements covering these dimensions with a 5-point scale for each item scored from 0 for 'strongly disagree' to 4 for 'strongly agree'. There is a maximum score of 200 indicating the ideal education environment as perceived by the student. Excellence is indicated by a score of 151–200.

Instruments have been developed to assess the education environment in postgraduate education (PHEEM), in the anaesthetic theatre (ATEEM) and in the surgery theatre (STEEM) (Roff 2005).

THE USE OF ENVIRONMENT MEASURES

Measurements of the education environment can be used to:

- establish the profile for an institution and gain a holistic view of the curriculum
- understand students' perceptions of the education environment they have experienced and compare it with their perception of the ideal environment
- compare the perceptions of the different stakeholders including staff, students and managers
- compare the environment as it exists in different departments or attachments within a school and at different phases of the training programme
- provide the medical school or postgraduate body, as a 'learning organisation', with an indication of what may be lacking in their programme and where change may be necessary, while at the same time nurturing aspects where no change is required
- assess the effect of a change made in the curriculum, comparing the education environment before and after the change
- compare the environment of different medical schools or geographical settings.

CONCLUSIONS

The education climate or environment is a key factor in the success of an undergraduate or postgraduate education programme. Measurement of the education environment provides valuable information relating to curriculum planning and evaluation. Quality assurance of education programmes involving all the stakeholders is on today's agenda. A pertinent and topical angle on this is the measurement of the education environment. Curriculum change may fail because changes have been made to the timetable, the teaching and learning methods and the assessment but without consideration being given to the education environment.

REFLECT AND REACT

1. Think about what type of learning environment you would wish to have as a student and how this compares with the environment that exists in your training programme.
2. If information is not already available, measure the education environment in your teaching situation using one of the tools available. On the basis of the results think about how the programme could be improved.
3. Reflect on how your own teaching and attitudes contribute to the education environment as perceived by students or trainees.

IF YOU HAVE A FEW HOURS

Genn, J.M., 2001. Curriculum, environment, climate, quality and change in medical education – a unifying perspective. AMEE Medical Education Guide. No. 23 Med. Teach. 23, 445–454 .
A key text on the subject that merits careful reading.

Hoff, T.J., Pohl, H., Bartfield, J., 2004. Creating a learning environment to produce competent residents: the roles of culture and context. Acad. Med. 79, 532–540.
Ideas from management theory helped the authors identify attitudes, behaviours and interactions that define a learning culture.

Holt, M.C., Roff, S., 2004. Development and validation of the Anaesthetic Theatre Educational Environment Measure (ATEEM). Med. Teach. 26, 553–558.
A description of how the measure was developed and how it is capable of identifying problem areas that can be remediated.

McAleer, S., Soemantri, D., Roff, S., 2009. Educational environment. In: Dent, J.A., Harden, R.M. (Eds.), A Practical Guide for Medical Teachers. third ed. Elsevier, London, pp. 64–70 (Chapter 9).

Roff, S., 2005. Education environment: a bibliography. Med. Teach. 27, 353–357.
A list of over 100 relevant articles.

Roff, S., McAleer, S., Harden, R.M., et al., 1997. Development and validation of the Dundee Ready Education Environment Measure (DREEM). Med. Teach. 19, 295–299.
The first description of this important inventory.

Roff, S., McAleer, S., Skinner, A., 2005. Development and validation of an instrument to measure the postgraduate clinical learning and teaching educational environment for hospital-based junior doctors in the UK. Med. Teach. 27, 326–331.
A description of the development of the Postgraduate Hospital Educational Environment Measure (PHEEM).

Shobhana, N., Wall, D., Jones, E., 2006. Can STEEM be used to measure the educational environment within the operating theatre for undergraduate medical students? Med. Teach. 28, 642–647.
The Surgical Theatre Educational Environment Measure was shown to be a reliable and practical tool for measuring the operating theatre educational environment.

Mapping the curriculum

A clear picture of how learning outcomes, teaching methods and student assessment link together is crucial not only for the teacher but also for the student. A curriculum map is needed.

Planning a curriculum is a complex matter involving learning outcomes, content, a timetable, the programme of teaching and learning opportunities and assessment. An aspect of curriculum development that has been relatively neglected is communication about the curriculum. How do teachers and students know what is covered and where it is addressed? How do students know what learning opportunities are available to assist them in mastering the learning outcomes? How does assessment relate to the teaching programme? Unfortunately students and trainees may perceive a curriculum or educational programme as a 'magical mystery tour' with the answer to these questions uncertain. They are not quite sure what lies ahead, or even about their destination, apart from the fact that they will end up with a qualification if they complete the course satisfactorily. The challenge is to communicate effectively to staff and students information about the curriculum. Curriculum mapping alongside a statement of the learning outcomes addresses the problem.

A curriculum map can provide information about what is taught, how it is taught, when it is taught, where it is taught and how the learning is assessed. It should be a key feature of any curriculum.

DEFINITION

A curriculum map is a visual representation of a curriculum that shows the big picture and how the different elements are related and linked together. It presents the curriculum as a sophisticated blend of educational strategies, course content, learning outcomes, educational experiences, assessment and programme of courses. It can even be thought of as the glue that holds the curriculum together. An example of part of a curriculum map through the window of learning outcomes is given in Figure 19.1.

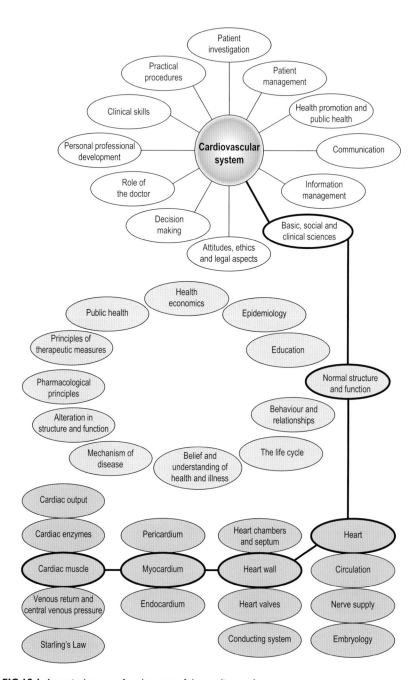

FIG 19.1 A curriculum map for elements of the cardiovascular system.

CURRICULUM MAPPING IS ON TODAY'S AGENDA

There are a number of reasons why the preparation of a curriculum map is now an essential element in planning and implementing a curriculum:

- **Outcome-based education.** The map makes explicit the expected learning outcomes for the different courses and learning experiences provided.

- **Student-centred learning.** The map of the curriculum helps students to take responsibility for their own learning, to appreciate what they are studying and the part it plays in the bigger picture, and how they can tailor the learning experiences to their personal needs.
- **Problem-based and integrated learning.** The map helps to clarify both the learning outcomes in PBL and integrated teaching programmes and the input from different disciplines.
- **Inter-professional education.** Common elements in the curriculum and the differences between medicine and other professions are described in a map. This facilitates the planning of inter-professional activities.
- **Integration of assessment and teaching.** The relationship between teaching and assessment is demonstrated in keeping with the move described in Section 5 towards 'assessment for learning'.
- **Distributed learning.** A map helps to ensure uniformity in the curriculum where this is delivered by a medical school on two or more sites.
- **Student mobility.** The transparency of the learning programme implicit in a curriculum map allows students' work to be recognised if they transfer to a different location. As envisaged in the Bologna process, a student may move on completion of the first cycle to complete the second cycle of their medical studies in another school.
- **The continuum of education.** A curriculum map assists the seamless transition between the different phases of undergraduate, postgraduate and continuing education and what is addressed in each phase.
- **Curriculum evaluation.** The curriculum map is of value for both internal and external assessment of the education programme including more formal accreditation and review by the public.
- **Changes in medicine.** A curriculum should be dynamic and not static in order that it can accommodate advances in medical practice. New subjects integrated into the curriculum are highlighted in the map. At the same time any redundancies and duplications in the curriculum can be recognised.

POTENTIAL USERS OF THE CURRICULUM MAP

The curriculum map may be of value to:

- **Teachers.** The map provides an overview of the curriculum programme in its entirety so that teachers can appreciate the place of their course within the curriculum and identify their own roles and responsibilities. Students or trainees frequently complain that incorrect assumptions are made by staff about what topics are covered elsewhere in the curriculum.
- **Curriculum planners.** The map provides a tool to assist the planner to evaluate the curriculum and keep it up-to-date. The map can be used to study whether what it is assumed the students are learning (the 'declared curriculum'), the curriculum that is presented (the 'delivered curriculum') and what students actually learn (the 'learned curriculum') are aligned.
- **Students.** The curriculum map together with the statement of expected learning outcomes and a study guide provide students with information that helps them to plan their programme of work and to assess their progress.

- **Administrators and support staff.** A curriculum map assists staff with the identification of resources necessary to implement the curriculum including staff, equipment and accommodation. It may also help to determine the contributions made by academic departments or individual members of staff to the curriculum and allow this to be recognised and rewarded.
- **Accrediting bodies.** The map may help to provide evidence that the medical school or postgraduate programme meets the expected requirements set out by accreditors.
- **Educational researchers.** There is a growing interest in research in medical education. The curriculum map is a useful tool for research into the existing curriculum or into changes made with regard to the teaching and assessment programme.

PREPARING A CURRICULUM MAP

Just for a moment put yourself in a different context. You are faced with planning a one-year's excursion to a part of the world with which you are unfamiliar. The first thing you need to inform your travel around the region is a map. This will show the different destinations and how each is located one to the other, the different transport options including roads, railways and airports, and the sites of objects of interest such as castles, lakes, etc. In much the same way a map of the curriculum includes:

- the expected learning outcomes
- the content, themes or topics addressed
- the learning experiences and resources available
- the assessment
- the courses and modules studied
- the timetable schedule.

The strength of the map lies in the links between these elements. For example, the learning outcomes, the learning experiences and the assessment are specified for each course or elements within a course or module. The maximum benefit is achieved through this multi-dimensionality with the ability to examine the curriculum from the perspective of any one element or window. For example, where in the curriculum is the communication skills learning outcome addressed; from the assessment perspective, where is professionalism evaluated; or what is the role of the clinical skills centre in the training programme?

Curriculum mapping has been limited by problems associated with storing, manipulating and updating the large amounts of information necessary and by the inability to view easily the information from different perspectives. The availability of electronic tools including multi-relational databases has given the concept of curriculum mapping a new impetus. Most schools that have developed a curriculum map, in the absence of suitable commercial software, have produced their own mapping programme.

The basis for a curriculum map may be a list of the courses or modules delivered over a period of time. To this can be added information about the learning outcomes, the learning experiences and the assessment of the course.

It may be helpful in the first instance in the preparation of a map to think about a series of two-dimensional matrices. For each learning opportunity timetabled event identified, the learning outcomes and the student assessment are specified.

REFLECT AND REACT

1. Think about how information relating to your curriculum is communicated to the students or trainees. To what extent is a map of the curriculum available that highlights for each part of the programme the learning outcomes, the learning opportunities and resources and the assessment procedures?
2. The investment of time necessary to map the curriculum can be rewarding and result in a much more powerful teaching and learning experience. Can you set some time aside to work on this?

EXPLORING FURTHER

IF YOU HAVE A FEW HOURS

Harden, R.M., 2001. Curriculum mapping: a tool for transparent and authentic teaching and learning. AMEE Guide No. 21 Med. Teach. 23, 123–137.
A description of curriculum mapping.

Ross, N., Davies, D., 1999. Outcome-based learning and the electronic curriculum at Birmingham Medical School. Med. Teach. 21, 26–31.
A description of an electronic curriculum map based on a database and delivered to staff and students via the web.

SECTION 4
FACILITATING LEARNING

'There can be no single way to study or best way to teach.'
Noel Entwistle. *Styles of Learning and Teaching*, 1981

OVERVIEW

Choose the most appropriate method from the rich menu of learning opportunities available and use it to maximum effect.

Chapter 20 The teacher's toolkit
There are many things to consider when choosing an educational tool from the wide range of instruments available. Think about the expected learning outcomes, the local context and the needs of the students.

Chapter 21 The lecture and teaching with large groups
Lectures can make a valuable contribution to the education programme. Careful consideration needs to be given to their role and how they are delivered.

Chapter 22 Learning in small groups
The advantages of small group teaching outweigh the problems that can arise. Conducted appropriately, small group sessions can be successful but be aware that the teacher's role should be one of facilitator.

Chapter 23 Independent learning
Students and trainees should be given more responsibility for their own learning. The learner may require support and direction.

Chapter 24 Teaching and learning in the clinical context
Lack of planning and feedback, coupled with poor supervision, often blights clinical teaching. The student, teacher and patient all have a role to play.

Chapter 25 Simulation of the clinical experience
Simulated patients, manikins, models and computer simulations complement experience with 'real' patients and have a place in a training programme.

Chapter 26 E-learning
The internet and resources available online have revolutionised medical education. They can make a significant contribution to your education programme.

Chapter 27 Peer and collaborative learning
Students learning from each other is effective. This can be informal or incorporated into scheduled activities.

The teacher's toolkit

There are many things to consider when choosing an educational tool from the wide range of instruments available. Think about the expected learning outcomes, the local context and the needs of the students.

CHOOSING A TEACHING METHOD

The FAIR educational principles (feedback, activity, individualisation and relevance) as described in Chapter 2, if applied in practice, result in effective learning. The creation of learning opportunities for students or trainees is the subject of this chapter.

The last decade has seen a re-examination of traditional teaching methods such as the lecture with a greater emphasis on small group work and independent learning, on the use of new learning technologies including simulation and e-learning and on learning in different contexts.

It is useful to think about the choice of teaching method from different perspectives:

- The expected learning outcomes. Learning outcomes, as argued in Chapter 6, should be the starting point in any consideration of teaching.
- The tools to be used, for example simulated patients or PowerPoint presentations.
- The context or location where the learning is situated, for example the lecture theatre, the outpatient clinic or the rural community.
- The educational strategies adopted in the curriculum or course, for example problem-based learning.
- Special needs of the trainees or students, for example do they have different starting points in their abilities or mastery of the subject?

LEARNING OUTCOMES

The choice of the most appropriate learning experience for students should take into account the expected learning outcomes. A lecture may be good for providing a framework or for transmitting information, but a small group discussion is more helpful if teamwork, reflection and problem solving are to be encouraged. Teaching in the clinical context, whether with real or simulated patients, can contribute to the acquisition of clinical skills as well as demonstrating relevance and the application of theory to practice.

125

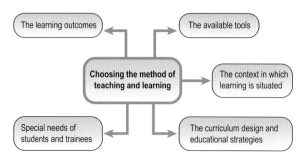

FIG 20.1 Choosing the method of teaching and learning.

Learning outcomes relating to patient safety, prevention of errors, team working, the promotion of health and the development of appropriate attitudes have been relatively neglected in the medical curriculum. The chapters that follow show how competence in these areas can be addressed if the appropriate teaching and learning method and the provision of appropriate learning opportunities are selected.

A blueprint or matrix should be prepared that matches the teaching and learning methods to the expected learning outcomes. The learning outcomes are placed on the horizontal axis and the learning methods or opportunities provided for students on the vertical axis. The vertical columns should identify at least one learning opportunity for each outcome. A learning opportunity can address several learning outcomes. Work with a simulated patient, for example, can cover both communication skills and attitude domains. A grid prepared in this way is useful not only in the planning of a training programme, but also for the students or trainees as a guide to their studies. The grid can be incorporated into a curriculum map or learning management tool if these are available.

THE TEACHER'S TOOLKIT

A competent carpenter or joiner has a toolkit with a range of tools, each of which has a key function for which it has been designed. A hammer is used to insert nails. Pliers could be used for the task but they are less efficient. The toolkit will include several types of saws, each suited to their own task. With time, the carpenter will replace old tools with new improved versions that incorporate the latest technology. If we employ a carpenter, we will expect him to have a comprehensive toolkit with the appropriate tools to tackle the job for which he has been engaged. Replace 'carpenter' with 'teacher' and the situation should be no different. The teacher should have a comprehensive up-to-date range of tools for teaching and learning. Students or trainees have the right to expect that we will incorporate in our teaching the methods most appropriate for the stated learning outcomes.

Tools available include:

- presentation tools such as PowerPoint to communicate ideas or principles particularly in a lecture context
- audience response systems (including simple coloured cards) to actively engage students in a lecture

- simulated patients and simulators to complement the use of real patients
- video clips to illustrate practical procedures
- podcasts or recordings of lectures
- games designed with an educational purpose
- online information sources and references
- computer-based learning opportunities such as virtual microscopy and interactive virtual patients
- networking tools such as Facebook to enhance collaborative learning
- peer-to-peer teaching where students support each other's learning.

An account of the tools available to the teacher is provided in the chapters that follow.

LEARNING CONTEXTS

Learning can take place in a range of contexts and situations – the classroom, the laboratory, the teaching hospital or the community. The most effective learning programmes offer a range of learning contexts with the appropriate mix or balance varying at different stages of training.

CLASSROOM CONTEXT

Classroom contexts include:

- **The lecture theatre.** Lectures have dominated many undergraduate courses. Their use and abuse are discussed later.
- **Small group work.** The value of small group teaching is now recognised along with the many advantages it offers. It is a key component of problem-based learning.
- **Practical laboratory or anatomy dissection room.** Traditional curricula provide learning opportunities in these locations. To some extent these have been replaced by alternatives including computer-based learning. (Methods used to teach anatomy are described in AMEE Guide No. 41 by Louw and co-workers (2009).)
- **Clinical skills centre.** Centres or laboratories with learning opportunities using simulators and simulated patients are a feature in many institutions. The importance of access to such facilities across all phases of education is now recognised.
- **Library, resource centre or computer suite.** The library today is very different from the library as we knew it in the past. It now includes a range of multi-media resources in addition to books. There is access to a computer, and often areas are set aside for students to learn together.

CLINICAL CONTEXT

Learning in the clinical context is at the very heart of medical education. There has been a move to more authentic learning relevant to medical practice, and the value of introducing students to patients from the first year of their studies has been demonstrated. A range of clinical contexts are available:

- **The hospital ward.** Traditionally this has provided the context for much of a student's clinical experience.

- **Ambulatory care.** With changes in hospital practice, ambulatory care and outpatient departments have provided an increasingly valuable component of a student's clinical experience.
- **Community.** Today there is increasing emphasis on community-based education in order to provide a broader perspective on patient care. The value of teaching and learning in the context of rural health care has been recognised.
- **Specialised settings**. Experience in more specialised settings such as palliative care or stroke units can provide valuable learning opportunities.

INFORMAL SETTINGS

Much of a student's education takes place away from the lecture theatre, the tutorial room or the clinic. Students may learn at home and informally from each other. Today's students are very different from those of previous generations. Networking and collaborative learning play an important part in their studies as described in Chapters 26 and 27.

EDUCATIONAL STRATEGIES

A range of educational strategies are described in Section 3. The strategy adopted has implications for the choice of learning method:

- In a *problem-based curriculum*, greater emphasis is usually (but not always) placed on small group work.
- In a *community-based curriculum*, learning takes place in a community, perhaps in a rural setting at a distance from the main education centre.
- In a *vertically integrated curriculum*, the use of simulations either in the form of simulated patients or simulators can introduce students effectively to clinical practice and practical procedures in the early years of their medical training.
- The use of a simulated ward may be valuable to support *inter-professional learning.*

Whatever educational strategy is adopted, it is likely that there will be a role for a range of teaching and learning methods. In problem-based learning, for example, while much of the emphasis will be on small group work and independent learning, the occasional lecture still has a place.

THE STUDENT OR TRAINEE

The learner should be kept sharply in focus when a learning method is selected. Think about:

- the number of students to be taught at any one time
- the background of the students and their individual needs
- the sophistication of the student in relation to new learning technologies
- the facilities available for independent learning.

Each student is different with regard to how their learning needs can best be met – one size does not fit all. As far as possible, their individual needs should be taken into account when the learning method is selected (see also Chapters 2 and 13). Not all students will choose to attend a lecture, and many may prefer an alternative approach.

Keep in mind that students are not simply the recipients of the training or educational programme. They may be co-authors and contribute actively to its development and delivery. This is discussed further in the section on peer teaching (Chapter 27).

Depending on the approach adopted the roles expected of the teacher will vary. There is likely to be a move away from the teacher as an information provider to one of learning facilitator.

A FINAL THOUGHT

While the emphasis in this section is on the range of teaching and learning methods and opportunities, an important element that contributes to the learner's success with any method is the teacher. The success or failure of an educational session will be related as much to how well it is planned and implemented by the teacher as to the choice of the learning approach. Different methods will make different demands on the teacher. Whatever the teacher's role, it needs to be fulfilled well if the learning is to be effective.

REFLECT AND REACT

Here are some thoughts to reflect upon in relation to your choice of teaching method:

1. There is no such thing as the single 'best' teaching method. Decide the best approaches for your students and trainees, taking into account the context and resources available.
2. Most teachers adopt teaching approaches with which they have gained experience and feel comfortable. Look again at your current approaches and consider whether you are using them to maximum effect. Are you sufficiently familiar with the range of methods available, including the new technologies such as simulation and e-learning, to allow you to make an informed decision about the best methods to be adopted in your situation? The descriptions in this book will assist you but it is particularly valuable if you can gain experience of the different approaches first hand at another centre or at an educational meeting. You should aim to harness in your teaching the best of new approaches alongside the best of existing proven methods.
3. Think about the different contexts in which the student or trainee can learn. Are you exploiting fully the range of contexts? In the undergraduate curriculum, for example, with the emphasis on more authentic learning, is sufficient emphasis being given in the early years to learning in the clinical setting and in the community? In the postgraduate curriculum, are sufficient opportunities provided for the trainee to work in a clinical skills centre or online?
4. Think about how you might offer a range of learning opportunities that match the needs of the individual student.

IF YOU HAVE A FEW HOURS

Ramsden, P., 2003. Learning to Teach in Higher Education, second ed. Routledge Falmer, London.
Chapter 9 in this useful book looks at teaching strategies for effective learning and develops further some of the issues raised in this chapter. It identifies problems associated with the choice of an appropriate teaching method.

IF YOU HAVE MORE TIME

Louw, G., Eizenberg, N., Carmichael, S.W., 2009. The Place of Anatomy in Medical Education. AMEE Guide No. 41. AMEE, Dundee.
A description of approaches to teaching anatomy.

McKeachie, W.J., 2010. Teaching Tips. Strategies, Research and Theory for College and University Teachers, twelfth ed. Houghton Mifflin Company, Boston.
The text, originally written to answer the questions posed by new teachers, highlights the decisions that need to be taken about the choice of teaching method.

The lecture and teaching with large groups

Lectures can make a valuable contribution to the education programme. Careful consideration needs to be given to their role and how they are delivered.

THE USE OF LECTURES

Of all the approaches to teaching, the lecture is perhaps the method most widely adopted. It is estimated that the average medical student sits through some 1800 lectures in the course of their studies. Most will be quickly forgotten. A few may be memorable. Despite much criticism, the lecture has stood the test of time. It has a lot to offer and should not be tossed aside as being ineffective and as a result excluded from the teacher's toolkit.

Brown and Manogue (2001) describe lectures as an economical and efficient method of conveying information to large groups of students. The lecture can provide an entrée into a difficult topic, it can offer different perspectives on a subject, it can communicate relevant personal, clinical or laboratory experience, and it can deliver a research-based view where teaching is immersed in a research-intensive university.

PROBLEMS WITH LECTURES

Problems attributed to the lecture may be the result of a 'bad lecturer' or the inappropriate use of the lecture. Common criticisms of lectures (Fig. 21.1) include:

- The lecture is a passive learning experience with a failure to engage the students in their own learning.
- Much of what is covered can be learned better from reading a book or engaging in an online programme.
- The delivery is difficult to follow with the visuals overloaded with information.
- The content of the lecture is inappropriate for the audience and is irrelevant, too advanced or too simple.

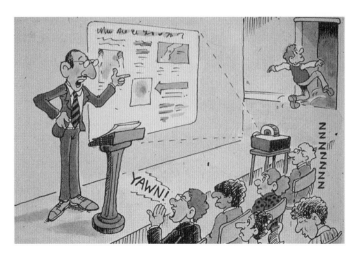

FIG 21.1   The lecture has been much criticised.

WHEN TO USE LECTURES

Lectures, if used properly, offer a number of advantages:

- The lecturer can meet simultaneously with a large group of students and convey his or her passion and enthusiasm for a subject.
- The lecture can serve as an introduction to a difficult topic and provide the students with a framework for their further studies.
- Dealing with a controversial area, the lecture can provide different perspectives and at the same time relate the topic to the local context.
- In an advancing area of knowledge, the lecture can provide up-to-date information and highlight the contributions of research in an area.
- The lecture can be used to provoke thought and discussion and to encourage the student to reflect on the topic.
- The lecture can include a practical demonstration, for example with a cardiac simulator or a patient introduced to illustrate a point (with the agreement of the patient).
- The lecture can provide the students with guidelines about their further study of the topic and can introduce the resources available.

DELIVERING A GOOD LECTURE

Lecturing can be a daunting task for some teachers who feel ill at ease when asked to perform in front of a large audience of students. Much of the stress can be alleviated with good planning and preparation.

GET SOME FACTS IN ADVANCE

Before concentrating on the content of the lecture, first do some fact finding:

- Refer to the statement of learning outcomes for the course. This should provide a clear idea of the purpose of the lecture and how it fits into the curriculum.
- Find out what the students already know about the subject of the lecture.

- Establish whether the lecture is one of a series of lectures on the subject and, if so, what the other lectures cover.
- Find out about the venue and the equipment to be used.

THINK ABOUT THE CONTENT AND STRUCTURE

Plan in advance the content and structure of the lecture:

- Plan the content for a lecture the students will wish to hear rather than the lecture you would like to give.
- Create a title for the lecture. It is sometimes easier to get started with the content if you first think of a title as it helps to structure your thoughts. It is more likely to interest students if the title is in the form of a question.
- Consider how you wish to structure the lecture. Two commonly used approaches are the classical method, where the lecture content is divided up into broad areas which are then subdivided, and the problem-centred approach where a problem or case study is presented and solutions are discussed. This chapter focuses on the classical approach although most of the tips given apply to both approaches.
- Lecturing styles vary considerably, so you must choose the style you feel most comfortable with and which suits your personality.

THE INTRODUCTION TO THE LECTURE

It is worth spending some time preparing your introduction. The first few minutes of the lecture are the most valuable. Try to instantly capture the attention of the audience and highlight why the content of the lecture is important. An engaging start to a lecture might include a press cutting of a case where an error has been made in the management of a patient, an illustration of a patient where an understanding of the pathophysiology proved valuable in the patient's management, or an interesting statistic highlighting the importance of the topic. Robert Cialdini is quoted as saying at the beginning of a lecture 'Here's a set of events unexplainable by common sense, and I promise you'll be able to solve this mystery at the end of the class'.

Don't keep the student in the dark about the content of the lecture. Tell the student what you are going to tell them, then tell them and finally tell them what you have told them. Advance organisers can help. These are signposts that help to guide the student through the content as you have structured it. For example, 'we will look in turn at six features of …' or 'first we will look at…then at…and finally at…'.

VISUAL AIDS

Visual aids help to reinforce and emphasise important points in a lecture and to explain difficult concepts or principles. They also help to vary the pace of the lecture and to maintain the student's interest. Video clips can be used to introduce case studies. Check for typographical errors on text visuals as spelling mistakes damage your credibility. Also make sure that students at the back of the lecture theatre will be able to read the text or captions on your visuals. It is amazing how many teachers fail to do this.

PowerPoint is an application designed to help the speaker or lecturer assemble professional looking slides and is widely used in oral presentations. The result sadly is often an unending stream of slides with bullet lists, animations that obscure rather than clarify the point and cartoons that distract from rather than convey the message. A host of sites are available on the web that provide practical advice on PowerPoint presentations and can help you to avoid 'death by PowerPoint' (Harden 2008).

Visual aids are a tool to help the teacher get a message across to students in the most effective way. The lecturer, not the PowerPoint slides, should be the star of the occasion. The text on slides should complement what is being said, not replace it.

TIPS ON LECTURING

It is normal for a lecturer to feel just a little bit anxious before a lecture. Have a glass of water at the podium or nearby just in case you 'dry up'. This will be less of a problem, however, if you have done the necessary preparation and have considered the following tips highlighted in the acronym 'LECTURE' (Fig. 21.2):

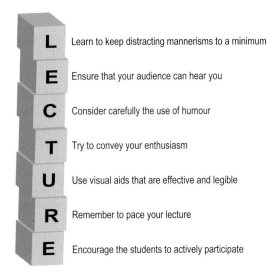

L Learn to keep distracting mannerisms to a minimum

E Ensure that your audience can hear you

C Consider carefully the use of humour

T Try to convey your enthusiasm

U Use visual aids that are effective and legible

R Remember to pace your lecture

E Encourage the students to actively participate

FIG 21.2 Hints on delivering a lecture.

- Learn to keep distracting mannerisms to a minimum – taking spectacles off and putting them back on or jingling coins can be annoying.
- Ensure that your audience, especially those at the back of the theatre or classroom, can hear you.
- Consider carefully the use of humour. Does it add to your lecture and can you really deliver the joke or cartoon or will your attempts fall flat?
- Try to convey your enthusiasm and passion for the subject. This will be almost impossible if you read your notes. You need to vary the volume, pitch and speed of your delivery.
- Use visual aids that are effective and are legible and be sure to rehearse with the equipment and lighting before the start of the lecture.

- **R**emember to pace your lecture and allow time for note-taking. Speaking at the rate of an express train will not go down well with students who are struggling to keep up.
- Encourage the students to actively participate in the lecture without them feeling inhibited or threatened and leave time at the end for questions or discussion. Some strategies for engaging the audience are described below.

ENGAGING THE AUDIENCE

There are a number of strategies that can be adopted to transform your presentation from a passive to an engaging and active experience for the student. These include:

- Introduce at various stages during the lecture questions on the subject with a number of alternative answers presented. Students are asked to respond using an electronic response system, or coloured cards can be used with a different colour corresponding to each answer.
- Incorporate mini brainstorming sessions during the lecture where groups of three, four or five students next to each other are encouraged to discuss a topic. Some groups are asked to report back to the whole class. Alternatively the groups may answer and respond to a multiple choice question using cards or an audience response system. This is a key activity in team-based learning.
- Introduce or build your presentation around a case study or patient management problem, involving the class as the problem develops.

THE CLOSE OF THE LECTURE

The close at the end of the lecture is almost as important as the introduction. Summarise the main concepts or messages you wish to convey and prepare the students for any further lectures that may follow in the series. Try also to leave students with something to think about which, following the lecture, may stimulate a discussion with their colleagues.

HANDOUTS

A handout of a lecture can provide the student with the framework and also the essential messages you wish to convey. It can be designed in such a way that students are encouraged to personalise it with their own notes as the lecture proceeds. Handouts may be valuable for revision purposes. Some lecturers use printed copies of their PowerPoint presentation as handouts but this is less satisfactory than handouts designed specifically for the purpose. If you want to encourage students to take notes, make sure that you leave sufficient time for this activity.

WHAT IS THE VERDICT?

Good teachers will evaluate their lectures. It is always helpful to receive feedback from students to ascertain the clarity of the presentation, the extent to which they found it interesting, and their perception of its relevance to the course and its value to them as an aid to their learning. An example of a questionnaire that can be used for this purpose is provided in Appendix 13. An additional insight into your lecture can be gained from inspecting the students' notes. Be warned! You might find the result a cause for concern.

A colleague may be invited to sit in the lecture and this peer assessment can provide an additional perspective on your performance. You can also assess your own performance if you have arranged for your lecture to be recorded.

REFLECT AND REACT

1. How would you rate your ability as a lecturer? What might you do to improve your performance?
2. Have you evaluated your performance from the perspective of your students or your peers?
3. What do you see as the main purpose of your lecture – to inform the students, to encourage them to reflect and think or to influence their attitudes to the subject?

EXPLORING FURTHER

IF YOU HAVE A FEW HOURS

Brown, G., Manogue, M., 2001. Refreshing lecturing: a guide for lecturers. AMEE Medical Education Guide No. 22. Med. Teach. 23, 231–244 .
This Guide provides an overview of the lecture, the processes of lecturing and suggestions for improvement.

Harden, R.M., 2008. Death by PowerPoint – the need for a 'fidget index'. Med. Teach. 30, 833–835.
Some practical hints on the use of PowerPoint in presentations.

Newman, L.R., Lown, B.A., Jones, R.N., et al., 2009. Developing a peer assessment of lecturing instrument: lessons learned. Acad. Med. 84, 1104–1110.
An interesting article which describes how an instrument was created for peer assessment of lecturing using a modified Delphi method.

O'Brien, T.E., Wang, W., Medvedev, I., et al., 2006. Use of a computerized audience response system in medical student teaching: its effect on exam performance. Med. Teach. 28, 736–738.
A description of the use of an audience response system in a haematology course at Case Western Reserve University School of Medicine, USA.

Robertson, L.J., 2000. Twelve tips for using computerised interactive audience response system. Med. Teach. 22, 237–239.

IF YOU HAVE MORE TIME

Bligh, D.A., 2000. What's the use of lectures? Jossey-Bass, San Francisco.
A classic text on the use of lectures.

Learning in small groups

The advantages of small group teaching outweigh the problems that can arise. Conducted appropriately, small group sessions can be successful but be aware that the teacher's role should be one of facilitator.

DEFINITION

Small group teaching has been a feature of education programmes for many years, particularly in the clinical context. With the introduction of problem-based learning (PBL) and team-based learning (TBL), small group teaching attracted renewed interest. Learners work together in a group, interacting with each other to achieve common learning goals. A tutor may facilitate the work of the group or it may be self-directed.

ROLE OF SMALL GROUP TEACHING

Small group teaching should be included in the teacher's tool kit as students working in small groups can master learning outcomes not readily achievable using other learning methods.

Learning outcomes achieved through small group teaching include:

- The development of social and interpersonal skills and communication skills such as listening and debating. These skills have been recognised as important learning outcomes to be addressed in an educational programme.
- The ability of a student to work as a member of a team and to recognise the roles of other team members. Students are encouraged in small group work to behave in a professional manner and to respect the views of others in the group. Doctors need to work effectively as team members and the skills that enable them to do so should not be taken for granted.
- The ability for students to engage in problem solving, critical thinking, the analysis of a complex issue and refining their understanding.
- The fostering of skills required by students to cope with uncertainty. This reflects medical practice where issues are frequently complex and uncertainty not uncommon.
- Innovative thinking, creativity and the development of new ideas.
- Deep learning with a more complete understanding of the subject rather than superficial learning where there is an emphasis on memorisation.

- Students reflecting on their own abilities and attitudes and exploring further the concept of professionalism in medical practice. Members of the group may find preconceived beliefs challenged.
- Students' ability to take responsibility for their own learning.

ADVANTAGES

In addition to achieving key outcomes as outlined above, small group work offers a number of possible advantages:

- Small group learning embraces the FAIR principles of effective learning as described in Chapter 2. In particular it encourages active rather than passive learning and provides learners with immediate feedback with regard to their understanding and attitude to a subject.
- Students find working in properly organised small groups engaging and motivating and are encouraged to continue further with the learning process. The approach does place demands on the students but they find the less formal atmosphere of group work more relaxed and conducive to learning. The experience may even be enjoyable.
- Small group work draws and builds on the expertise and talents of the members of the group. The less effective and efficient learners may learn from others in the group and improve their learning skills. Studies have shown that where a number of groups are addressing a problem, the results from the 'poorest' group are invariably better than the results from the best individual student working alone.

PROBLEMS WITH SMALL GROUP TEACHING

This approach to teaching can be problematic. Teachers may not use the method effectively and some group sessions are mismanaged:

- Teachers accustomed to lecturing may be less experienced in the role of facilitator in the small group setting. As a result, small group work deteriorates into mini lectures.
- Small group teaching is considerably more difficult to manage than a lecture as more attention needs to be paid to individual students' behaviour, personalities and difficulties. Diversity in a group promotes varied and interesting opinions, but it also has the potential to create conflict and may interfere with the proper functioning of the group.
- Scheduling the necessary number of rooms for small group teaching may present a logistical problem. If a class of 180 students has small group activities scheduled at the same time with nine students in a group, 20 small group rooms need to be made available. This is not a problem in team-based learning as the small group activities take place in a lecture theatre or large demonstration room.
- Excessive demands may be placed on teachers' time requiring a higher than normal teacher–student ratio. This can be less of a problem if there is a greater emphasis placed on student-directed groups, or if one teacher, as in the team-based learning approach, manages a number of small groups.

- Students too often are not briefed before a small group session as to the benefits to be gained and the expected learning outcomes. This can result in them being less favourably disposed to the teaching method. They may not value what they learn in the small group work and may consider it to be a less effective use of their time when compared to attending a lecture or reading a textbook.

TECHNIQUES USED IN SMALL GROUP WORK

A number of approaches can be used to organise a small group session. Some will be more applicable than others, depending on the situation, the learners, the local context and the expected learning outcomes:

- **Brainstorming.** This is a creative thinking exercise in which group members generate as many ideas as possible without criticising or questioning their validity until time or ideas are exhausted. The ideas are then discussed. This approach is especially valuable to encourage creativity and generate new ideas.
- **Snowballing.** Learners work initially in pairs to discuss the issue or task. They then join with another pair to compare and contrast their results. The group of four learners then combines with another group of four and the exercise is repeated. The deliberations are finally discussed in a plenary session. Snowballing particularly encourages clarification of ideas and values in a non-threatening situation. A variation of snowballing is the jigsaw group. With this technique, after a topic is discussed, the groups reform into new groups, with each new group containing one member of the old group.
- **Role-playing.** Students enact a scenario assuming in turn the role of the doctor, nurse or patient. Role-playing is particularly valuable in exploring communication issues and attitudes. The sessions may be videotaped and this can be helpful to students who can view and analyse their own performance and learn from it.
- **Journal club.** This approach is frequently used in postgraduate education. Participants are asked to present and comment on recent papers in the medical literature. The group then discusses the comments.
- **Tutorial/seminar.** Tutorials are particularly helpful to enable students to critically probe subject matter in more detail. This helps them to clarify and expand on their understanding. Triggers such as clinical photographs, a videotape clip or a short student presentation may be used as a springboard for the tutorial. In a tutorial, the group can discuss material that has been covered in a lecture or in a directed self-learning exercise. The tutorial may be focused on aspects of the subject where students have encountered difficulties.
- **Problem-based learning.** Small group work plays a key role in PBL as discussed in Chapter 14. Group discussions are directed around a problem presented to the group. The students' learning needs relating to the problem are identified.
- **Clinical teaching.** Teaching is conducted with a small number of students around patients in the ward or outpatient department. Clinical skills centres also provide the setting for clinical teaching with small groups using simulated patients and models. Clinical teaching is discussed in more detail in Chapter 24.

THE ROLE OF THE TEACHER

It is obvious from these descriptions that small group activities can take many different forms. The way in which students engage in group work and the role of the teacher will vary. The approaches can be placed on a continuum from student centred to teacher centred and the role of the teacher will vary accordingly. At the 'teacher-centred' end of the spectrum, the small group session consists of a seminar or tutorial or bedside teaching with the teacher in the role of the information provider. There is likely, however, to be more student interaction than can be found in a lecture situation. At the student-centred end of the spectrum, the teacher's role is one of facilitating the group. The group may even be student led. The role of the teacher in the small group falls into one or more of the following categories:

- chair person – eliciting information and opinions from the group and managing the group process
- consultant – providing information or specialist knowledge in an area
- observer – commenting on the group discussion at appropriate places
- devil's advocate – confronting and challenging the group
- counsellor – releasing tensions in the group where members feel threatened or where some students dominate the discussions.

Facilitating a small group is one of the most skilled tasks the teacher can undertake. The teacher has to guide the work of the group and encourage the learners to interact. At the same time he or she must guard against dominating the group.

There has been much discussion, particularly in the context of PBL, as to whether the group facilitator should be a content expert or a person who has the facilitating skills without necessarily having content expertise. In most situations content expertise is seen as an important prerequisite for the teacher. This is particularly so in bedside teaching where one role of the teacher is that of information provider. Content expertise on its own, however, is insufficient and it is important that a teacher has an understanding of the small group process and the necessary facilitation skills.

Some teachers are better than others at running small group sessions and some medical schools or postgraduate institutions prefer only to use as group facilitators teachers who excel in this area. There should be a staff development programme in place to help teachers learn the skills involved.

IMPLEMENTING SMALL GROUP WORK

A number of tasks have to be carried out at each stage of a small group session.

BEFORE A SMALL GROUP ACTIVITY

A small group activity may appear relatively informal but to be effective it has to be well planned. The teacher needs to:

- Decide which approach to small group work will be adopted and the types of small group activities to be included. For example, will there be an element of brainstorming or snowballing?
- Determine the number of students in the group and the composition. Group size can vary but a generally accepted optimum number of

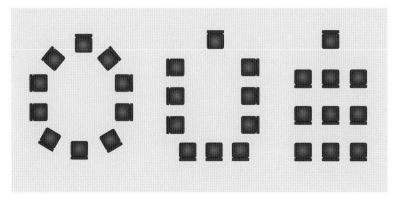

FIG 22.1 Scenarios of a seating plan for small group teaching.

students is seven or eight. In some situations this has to be expanded but should probably never exceed 12.

- Arrange the venue for the group meeting and the seating arrangements in a way that will encourage discussion. Figure 22.1 shows three scenarios. The first is the preferred option and maximises the interaction of the group. The second emphasises the role of the teacher or group leader. The third replicates a lecture theatre setting and should be avoided.
- Create the right learning environment. For example, noise from adjacent rooms can be a distracter.
- Consider and specify the expected learning outcomes of the session. These will reflect both the subject matter or theme for the group session and also more generic competencies such as reflection and interpersonal skills.
- Plan the necessary resources, e.g. trigger material in the form of a short video clip, case study or published paper. In the clinical context there are real or simulated patients.
- Brief the students in advance if you expect them to do some preparatory work or gain practical experience in the area prior to the small group session.

DURING A SMALL GROUP ACTIVITY

There is no one best way of managing a small group and dealing with any problems as they arise. The following guidelines may be helpful:

- The group members should introduce themselves to each other and state their personal goals and expectations. This sets the scene for the work to be done.
- Review the expected learning outcomes and how these will be achieved. Students may enter the small group activity with some reluctance, feeling the time spent is wasteful and that they will learn better in some other way. One of the common reasons for groups failing is the lack of clear goals and outcomes.

- Establish the ground rules for working as a group, recognising that some people may feel threatened in the group situation. Rules should ensure that contributions are received positively. A typical rule might be that only one member talks at any one time and that all members contribute.
- Create a positive atmosphere for the students' learning. There has to be an atmosphere of mutual trust and respect and they should feel comfortable enough to expose their areas of weakness.
- Focus the group on the task in hand. How this is done will depend on the agreed learning outcomes and group methods adopted. Keep the learning process moving.
- Encourage participation from members of the group by using open-ended questions, listening to what is being said and responding. Monitor the progress of each student in the group.
- Avoid being the centre or focus of the small group activity and do not provide information that other members of the group can provide or that they can get elsewhere.
- Keep the discussion at the appropriate level. It should not be boring or over-challenging.
- Recognise the different roles group members play, for example information provider or influencer, and use this information to help the group accomplish the task.
- Tackle problems in the group, such as a dominant, garrulous or lazy learner, by calling 'time out' and asking the group how they want to solve the issue.
- Towards the end of the session summarise what has been achieved and plan what is expected of the group before they next meet.

AFTER THE SMALL GROUP ACTIVITY

After a small group session be sure to:

- Support any follow-up actions identified at the group meeting. This may include access to further learning opportunities or communication online between group members.
- Plan any further small group sessions if required.
- Complete any student attendance sheets or student evaluation required.
- Evaluate the small group session, for example through student feedback forms. Reflect on the experience gained by the students and yourself, and consider how the small group session might be improved if it has to be repeated.

REFLECT AND REACT

1. Are you making sufficient use of small group methods in your teaching programme?
2. If you are using or considering using small group teaching, look again at the learning outcomes you expect your learners to achieve. How do these compare with the suggested outcomes for small group work described above?

3. Which small group methods would be appropriate in your own context and what is your role in the group?
4. Would attending a staff development programme on small group teaching be helpful to you?

EXPLORING FURTHER

IF YOU HAVE A FEW HOURS

Edmunds, S., Brown, G., 2010. Effective Small Group Learning. AMEE Guide No. 48. AMEE, Dundee.
An overview of the use of small group methods in medicine and what makes them effective.

Crosby, J.R., Hesketh, E.A., 2004. Developing the teaching instinct: 11: Small group learning. Med. Teach. 26, 16–19.
A brief guide to the use of small group learning in medicine.

McCrorie, P., 2010. Teaching and leading small groups. In: Swanwick, T. (Ed.), Understanding Medical Education: Evidence, Theory and Practice. Wiley-Blackwell, Chichester.
A useful introduction to the use of small group work in medical education.

Steinert, Y., 1996. Twelve tips for effective small-group teaching in the health professions. Med. Teach. 18, 203–207.
Practical suggestions for successfully implementing small group learning.

IF YOU HAVE MORE TIME

Miflin, B., 2004. Small groups and problem-based learning: are we singing from the same hymn sheet? Med. Teach. 26, 444–450.
Small group learning considered in the context of PBL.

Independent learning

Students and trainees should be given more responsibility for their own learning. The learner may require support and direction.

In Chapters 21 and 22 we looked at how students learn in the lecture and small group settings. Independent learning by students outside these contexts has always been a feature of education. The importance of independent learning, where students take charge of their learning and tailor it to their own particular needs, has become increasingly recognised.

THE IMPORTANCE OF INDEPENDENT LEARNING

There are a variety of reasons for the increased interest in independent learning:

- There has been a move from teacher-centred learning, where the emphasis is on what the teacher teaches, to student-centred learning with the emphasis on what the student learns.
- The excessive use of lectures as a learning experience has been criticised and more time is available in the curriculum for other learning activities.
- Curricula now include electives or options where, for part of the course, students plan their own studies as described in Chapter 17.
- Collaborative learning and peer-to-peer learning is increasingly becoming part of mainstream education as discussed in Chapter 27.

THE BENEFITS OF INDEPENDENT LEARNING

Independent learning offers a number of advantages:

- With a more diverse student population now admitted to medical school, the learning can be matched to the needs of the individual student.
- The move to an outcome-based model (see Section 2) has made it easier for students to understand what is expected of them and makes it possible for them to create their own personal learning programme. When asked about the necessity of attending lectures students indicate that the main reason is to learn what they should be studying. In outcome-based education the learning outcomes are transparent.
- There is an increasing focus on distance learning and hybrid models that incorporate face-to-face and distance learning. Independent learning by the student is a key feature.

- Students now learn in a variety of sites such as the community, the district hospital and clinical skills centres. This often results in the students having to take more responsibility for their own learning.
- The need for life-long learning and continuing professional development is recognised. This requires students to learn to take more responsibility for their own learning early in their training and to acquire and refine the necessary learning skills.
- Advances in technology and internet developments have resulted in rich and powerful learning experiences becoming available.
- If independent learning is used to replace some lectures, the teacher is free to engage in more rewarding activities interacting with small groups or individual students.

BENEFITS FOR THE STUDENT

When compared to the more formal lecture or small group setting, independent learning offers the student a number of advantages. Students can:

- Choose to work at their own pace spending whatever time is necessary to achieve the required mastery of the subject.
- Decide when and where they study. This may be in the work place, on the job or at home.
- Tailor the content of the learning to their personal learning needs.
- Select the method of learning and an instructional design to match how they best learn. Some students are visual learners while others prefer the audio channel.
- Engage to a greater extent in deep learning and reflect on the subject as they pursue their studies.
- Monitor their own progress, using appropriate learning resources, and adjust their continuing learning based on feedback received.

ROLE OF INDEPENDENT LEARNING IN THE CURRICULUM

Two questions have to be asked about the role of independent learning in the curriculum. First, how much time should be scheduled in the curriculum for independent learning or private study? Some curricula have formal activities timetabled from 9.00am until 5.00pm leaving the student free for independent study only at other times. This is built on the premise that if time is left for private study students will not make full use of the opportunity and teachers will not be employed in the work for which they have been engaged. A second question relates to the extent to which the students' independent learning should be managed or the control left with the students. There are strong arguments for replacing the term 'self-directed learning' with the term 'directed self learning' as all students benefit from some direction or management of their learning. The need for this will vary from student to student, and with the same student in the different phases of undergraduate and postgraduate education. It has been suggested that the level of autonomy given to a student is one of the most important decisions a teacher has to make. Too little direction will result in confusion and inefficient and ineffective learning. Excessive direction will be demotivating and even result in boredom. This is described in Chapter 13.

THE ROLE OF THE TEACHER

The teacher's role in independent learning is very different from that to which he or she may be accustomed. There is a switch in emphasis from the teacher as the information provider to the teacher as the facilitator of the student's learning. The role of facilitator is a more demanding one and requires an appreciation of the needs of the learners and the potential problems the students may encounter when working on their own. A teacher is responsible for:

- Creating a supportive learning environment for students that encourages independent learning, self-confidence, curiosity and the desire to continue to learn. Independent learning will be fostered by a climate that is flexible and responsive to the learner's needs.
- Briefing students on the role of independent learning in the curriculum and, if students are relatively inexperienced, providing counselling and advice on the skills required.
- Working with the students to help them develop their own learning plan.
- Communicating the core learning outcomes expected of the student.
- Assisting students to identify appropriate learning resource materials and providing advice on how they can best be used. The teacher may also create new learning materials or annotate or adapt existing resources.
- Advising and assisting students to monitor their progress and assess their mastery of the subject.
- Responding to problems that may arise and being available, perhaps at a specified time and place, to advise students.

LEARNING RESOURCES

A wide range of learning resources are available to support independent learning. These include:

- Published books and journal articles. Print has the advantage that it does not require technology. It is highly portable, and the text can be easily annotated or highlighted.
- DVDs. These have the advantage of offering multi-media images including video clips of procedures or personal commentaries from the author.
- Online resources. An increasing amount of learning material is available for instant access through a range of websites including YouTube, Wikipedia and Facebook. There may be a problem however with quality assurance.
- Recordings and podcasts of lectures.
- Resources delivered through smart phones and other mobile devices such as the iPad.
- Tele- and web-conferences using a tool such as Wimba. These allow live interaction with other students and with a teacher or facilitator.
- Models and simulators as discussed in Chapter 25.
- Patients, both real and simulated, as discussed in Chapter 25.

The choice of learning resources will depend on the expected learning outcomes, the resources available and the technology support.

A teacher may wish to create independent learning resources for use by his or her students. Unless these are simply recordings of their teaching sessions, which is not advised, it can be a demanding task and is best undertaken in collaboration with an educational technologist or a colleague who has experience in the technology and in instructional design. The same general educational principles apply that were described in Chapter 2. Feedback should be provided, learning should be active rather than passive, and the students encouraged to reflect on what they have learned. Students should be able to individualise the resources to meet their own personal needs and the content should be relevant and matched to the specified learning outcomes.

INDEPENDENT LEARNING AND THE CURRICULUM

Independent learning can be scheduled in the curriculum:

- As a replacement for scheduled activities such as lectures. It may be used as a substitute for lectures when a new course is planned or to replace lectures in an existing course to free students' time for other activities.
- As an alternative option to student attendance at a lecture. Podcasts are available for this purpose in many medical schools. Students have the choice of attending the lecture or covering the topic at a time and place more convenient to them.
- As an adjunct to existing learning opportunities. The modern equivalent of the reading list includes URLs for online resources and other multimedia. The teacher can provide annotations and comments to assist the student to select the most appropriate resources.
- For revision or remedial purposes.

STUDY GUIDES

The concept of study guides to support a student's learning was introduced in Chapter 13. They can play an important part in independent learning. The student is guided through the range of learning opportunities and given advice on how they can make the best use of the available time. The guide can include activities relating to the topic.

Guides can be provided in printed or electronic format. An extract from a study guide for junior doctors is shown in Appendix 4. Icons and the page layout are used to facilitate learning. The design of a study guide varies depending on how it is intended the student will make use of it. The position of a study guide on the study guide triangle (Fig. 23.1) indicates the extent to which the guide has been designed to:

- help students to manage their learning
- suggest activities to facilitate the learning
- provide content to support the student's learning.

A guide can be positioned anywhere on the study guide triangle, depending on its intended use.

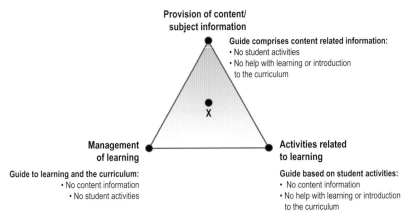

FIG 23.1 The study guide triangle with the three extremes identified and a guide with an equal emphasis on content provision, management of learning and activities represented at X.

DISTANCE LEARNING

Some institutions have gone as far as putting complete courses or modules online. A student may be able to complete a course of study almost entirely at a distance from the course provider. It is more usual for a hybrid model to be adopted that blends independent learning and face-to-face elements.

Students working independently have a choice of when and where they study (Fig. 23.2). This may be at a central learning resource centre on campus, in a peripheral training facility at a distance from the teacher and the main campus, or at home. In synchronous learning the time is fixed and students interact live with other students or with the teacher. A typical example of this is a telephone or web-conference or an online chat room. Working asynchronously, students may choose the time at which they wish to learn and communicate with other students and the teacher. This may be done using email or bulletin boards.

Time		
Varied	Learning resource centre	Asynchronous distance learning
Fixed	Classroom face-to-face meeting	Synchronous distance learning
	Fixed	Fixed	**Place**

FIG 23.2 In distance learning the place and time of learning may be fixed or varied.

PROBLEMS WITH INDEPENDENT LEARNING

Independent learning has an important role to play in undergraduate, post-graduate and continuing education. Problems can arise if it is left to chance, if insufficient preparatory work is done or if there is a lack of guidance and support for the students to allow them to make the best use of the time available.

REFLECT AND REACT

The task of planning the student's or trainee's independent learning is a significant responsibility.

1. Consider whether you have the right balance in your teaching programme between face-to-face contact with your students and opportunities for students to work on their own. Is time scheduled in the curriculum for independent learning?
2. Do you do enough to help the students maximise the benefits of learning on their own through the provision of advice and/or study guides to support the students' learning?
3. Are the benefits to be gained from the use of the new technologies sufficiently exploited in your programme?
4. Consider the level of autonomy that you offer the student and the control that you exert over their learning. How does this change as the student progresses through the course?
5. Consider whether you might work on the creation of learning resource material and if so with whom you might collaborate.

EXPLORING FURTHER

IF YOU HAVE A FEW HOURS

Harden, R.M., Laidlaw, J.M., Hesketh, E.A., 1999. Study guides: their use and preparation. AMEE Guide No. 16. Med. Teach. 21, 248–265.

Montemayor, L.L.E., 2002. Twelve tips for the development of electronic study guides. Med. Teach. 24, 473–478.

IF YOU HAVE MORE TIME

Dron, J., 2007. Control and Constraint in e-Learning: Choosing When to Choose. IDEA Group Publishing, London.
A useful discussion of how much autonomy should be given by the teacher to the student to manage their learning.

Laidlaw, J.M., Hesketh, E.A., Harden, R.M., 2009. Study guides. In: Dent, J.A., Harden, R.M. (Eds.), A Practical Guide for Medical Teachers. third ed. Elsevier, London (Chapter 27).,
This chapter outlines important trends in independent learning.

Teaching and learning in the clinical context

Lack of planning and feedback, coupled with poor supervision, often blights clinical teaching. The student, teacher and patient all have their role to play.

DEFINITION

Clinical teaching is teaching that focuses on real patients in clinical settings. The setting may be the hospital ward, out-patient department or surgical theatre, or the community.

CHANGING PERCEPTIONS OF CLINICAL TEACHING

Clinical teaching should be at the heart of medical education but how it is delivered is sadly often ignored. Traditionally the training of a doctor was based on the apprenticeship model where the trainee was attached to a reputable physician and worked with the physician in the day-to-day care of patients. This approach provided a relevant and practical training but had two disadvantages. There was a perceived lack of scientific underpinning of

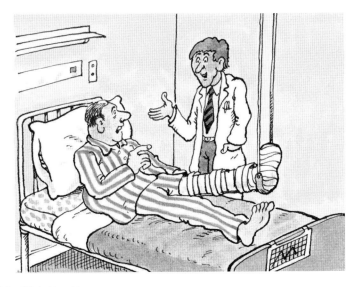

FIG 24.1 Clinical teaching.

the education and the quality of the training varied with the trainer's capacity and conscientiousness. For these reasons, as described earlier in the book, in the early part of the twentieth century training was moved to medical schools and associated with a defined curriculum. A greater emphasis was put on the scientific basis for medicine and this played a key role in the early training of a doctor and lectures were widely adopted. In the past two decades there has been a move to return an emphasis in training to the clinical context, with the provision of authentic learning experiences from the early years of the undergraduate curriculum. Changes have also taken place in postgraduate education with the recognition that the education of the trainee does not need to conflict with his or her service role in the delivery of health care. With an appropriate curriculum and planning, learning can be managed 'on the job' in the context of the trainee's work.

THE IMPORTANCE OF CLINICAL TEACHING

The advantages of clinical training are obvious:

- If it is implemented appropriately, students are motivated by the relevance of the learning. Students enter medicine to become doctors, and learning with patients and from patients is a powerful and effective learning experience.
- Learning round a patient helps to convey a holistic approach to medical care that combines the necessary knowledge, skills and attitudes.

THE STUDENT

Key players in clinical teaching are the student, the teacher and the patient. The role of the student in the clinical setting varies depending on their seniority and their stage in the curriculum. A junior student may actively engage in learning while not being a member of the team delivering the patient's care. Students may visit the ward in groups of six to ten and be taught on one or more selected patients by an assigned clinical teacher. Students observe the teacher taking a patient's history or examining the patient and may have the opportunity to do so themselves. The students are then questioned on the findings and required to reflect on the patient's case. Feedback is given to the student.

A more senior student participates in a clerkship as a member of the health-care team. The teaching is integrated into the care of the patient. Students move from a peripheral role to one of participating as members of the medical community of practice. Students learn from working alongside experienced practitioners and other members of the healthcare team. In the process they are socialised into the practice of medicine. The ward round and patient care conferences are typical learning opportunities.

In postgraduate training, work-based learning is the norm with the trainees developing their competencies as junior members of the healthcare team with certain assigned responsibilities. Short courses relating to specialised aspects of the work or procedures can be scheduled.

THE TEACHER

The role of the clinical teacher is particularly challenging as it encompasses the range of roles highlighted in Chapter 1. These include information provider, role model, facilitator, mentor, assessor and planner. Clinical teachers assume multiple roles when they interact with their students. They need to be 'the expert' and a source of knowledge while at the same time facilitating the students' learning by having an understanding about the teaching and learning process. Both senior and junior doctors serve as role models for students. Many studies have explored the attributes of a good clinical teacher and these are summarised in Table 24.1.

Table 24.1 *Features of the good clinical teacher*

Good clinical teacher	Bad clinical teacher
Plans the clinical teaching with clearly defined learning outcomes	Haphazard approach with no clear plan
Appears enthusiastic with a positive attitude	Disinterested and regards the teaching as an intrusion into other commitments
Serves as a positive role model demonstrating good relationships with patients	Serves as a poor role model lacking aspects of professionalism in practice
Helpful and available to students	Intimidating and teaches by humiliation
Encourages student active participation	Didactic with student's role passive
Patient-orientated with problem solving	Disease-orientated and factual
Observes student examining patient and provides feedback	Listens to or reads students' reports of examination of patient and provides inadequate feedback
Provides students with opportunity to practise their skills	Does not encourage students to practise their skills
Tailors the teaching to the stage of training of the students and to the needs of the individual students	Does not take into consideration the stage of training of the students or their individual needs

The skills required of a clinical teacher too often have been taken for granted and it has been assumed that if doctors are good practitioners, they are also good teachers. Unfortunately deficiencies and poor practice in clinical teaching have been widely recognised. Problems identified include the lack of planning, inappropriate supervision, lack of feedback and failure to appreciate basic educational principles as to how students learn.

THE PATIENT

Clinical teaching is unique as the key element is the patient. The patient may be a hospital in-patient or out-patient or may be located in the community. In addition to learning with 'real patients', students can benefit from exposure to simulations including simulated patients, manikins and computer representations as described in Chapter 25. These tools can complement but not replace experience with real patients. Patients locate the teaching in the real world, provide more authentic learning experiences and help to ensure that the teaching is relevant. Patients as well as the teacher can provide feedback to the student about their techniques, attitude and communication skills.

The range of patients seen by students in a clinical attachment should reflect the expected learning outcomes. This can be recorded in a portfolio and any gaps identified in a student's clinical experience should be remedied. Students who use an electronic hand-held device to document their patient encounters do so more completely. Patients can be selected for clinical teaching on the basis of their presenting problems, their availability and their willingness and ability to cooperate with the teaching programme. It is important to obtain full patient consent before students interact with the patients and it is important that the patient's comfort and dignity are respected. Patients may feel they have benefited from the experience.

PLANNING

As with all teaching approaches, planning is important. The expected learning outcomes must be clearly defined and communicated to the student. These may include skills in history taking, mastery of practical procedures and an understanding of ethical issues.

Appropriate learning opportunities, both formal and informal, should be scheduled in the learner's work plan. Teachers responsible for a formal teaching session should make arrangements for someone to cover their other commitments so that they are not interrupted by bleeps or other calls.

IMPLEMENTING

In a formal clinical teaching session students should be actively involved and engaged. They should feel free to ask questions and ask for help if required. They should be encouraged to reflect and think about the patients they see. Students can be helped to do this by the use of skilful questioning by the teacher, the aim of which includes:

- Arousing the learner's interest, e.g. 'How often do you think a general practitioner will see a patient with a thyroid problem?'
- Testing the learner's knowledge of the subject, e.g. 'Is this a reliable indicator that the patient is hyperthyroid?'
- Promoting the student's understanding and encouraging the student to reflect on the topic and stimulate their critical thinking, e.g. 'Which of the treatment options available would you advise in this case and for what reason?'
- Encouraging the learner to relate theory to practice: 'What is the explanation for the patient's tachycardia?'
- Inviting comparisons or different viewpoints, e.g. 'What is different in this patient from the last patient we saw?'
- Consolidating the learning through encouraging the trainee to review and summarise the learning that has occurred, e.g. 'What have you learned today from the experience?'

As a teacher you need to learn to be comfortable with silence. Give the students at least three to five seconds to think between asking a question and expecting an answer. Insufficient attention is paid to the art of questioning in staff development programmes. We have found the skill lacking even in experienced teachers.

As well as questioning the learner, it is important for the teacher also to be a good listener. You need to hear and understand what is being said and respond accordingly. Non-verbal behaviours are also important so try to maintain eye contact with the student.

In clinical teaching the provision of feedback to the learner is of particular importance. Feedback is an essential part of the learning process. It provides students and trainees with information about their performance and how they can improve upon it. It needs to be given skilfully if you want to motivate your students. The feedback should be timely, descriptive rather than evaluative, and specific rather than general. Try to provide positive suggestions and not just negative comments. This is discussed further in Chapter 2.

CLINICAL SUPERVISION

In postgraduate training programmes, the clinical supervisor provides the trainee with guidance and feedback on matters of personal, professional and educational development in the context of the provision of safe and appropriate patient care. Clinical supervision is important, but how it is carried out is highly variable. The clinical supervisor is responsible for:

- finding out the aspirations and career intentions of the trainee
- recognising the strengths and weaknesses of the trainee and adapting the training to the trainee's needs
- meeting regularly with the trainee to discuss the expected learning outcomes
- monitoring the trainee's progress and giving frequent and constructive feedback
- encouraging the trainee to be reflective by keeping a diary or portfolio of the clinical cases encountered
- being available to the trainee when support or advice is required
- offering counselling to the trainee if the need arises
- keeping the trainee motivated by being positive yourself
- keeping their personal knowledge base and practice up-to-date.

REFLECT AND REACT

1. Think about how you can ensure that your students or trainees achieve the expected learning outcomes when so much of their clinical experience is opportunistic.
2. Is sufficient care taken to inform and obtain consent from patients who participate in the clinical teaching and are they asked for feedback?
3. Do you adequately monitor the progress of students or trainees for whom you are responsible and provide them with frequent and constructive feedback?

IF YOU HAVE A FEW HOURS

Dolmans, D.H.J.M., Wolfhagen, I.H.A.P., Essed, G.G.M., et al., 2002. The impacts of supervision, patient mix, and numbers of students on the effectiveness of clinical rotations. Acad. Med. 77, 332–335.
The effectiveness of clinical rotations depends on high quality student supervision.

Dornan, T., Littlewoods, S., Margolis, S.A., et al., 2007. How Can Experience in Clinical and Community Settings Contribute to Early Medical Education? A BEME Systematic Review. BEME Guide No. 6. AMEE, Dundee.
Evidence as to the value of clinical experiences early in the curriculum.

Irby, D.M., Papadakis, M., 2001. Does good clinical teaching really make a difference? Am. J. Med. 110, 231–232.

Ramani, S., Leinster, S., 2008. Teaching in the clinical environment. AMEE Guide 34. Med. Teach. 30, 347–364.
An overview of clinical teaching with practical guidelines.

Spencer, J., 2010. Learning and teaching in the clinical environment. In: Cantillon, P., Wood, D. (Eds.), ABC of Learning and Teaching in Medicine, second ed. John Wiley and Sons, Chichester (Chapter 8).
A short overview of clinical teaching.

Sutkin, G., Wagner, E., Harris, I., et al., 2008. What makes a good clinical teacher in medicine? A review of the literature. Acad. Med. 83, 452–466.
A description of what is known about the attributes of a good clinical teacher.

Simulation of the clinical experience

Simulated patients, manikins, models and computer simulations all complement experience with 'real' patients and have a place in a training programme.

The importance of learning in the clinical context was emphasised in the previous chapter. A key element in clinical teaching is the patient. There is now good evidence that exposure to the 'real patient' can be augmented usefully with a simulated experience. Simulated patients and patient manikins or models are widely used and have been found to be of value in undergraduate education and postgraduate training to complement the student's experience with real patients. Some teachers have been sceptical about the use of simulation in medicine but its value is now proved. Simulation should be seen as a prelude to doing the real thing on a real patient, never as an end in itself.

In this chapter we look at different types of simulation, the educational strategies that need to be adopted and the concept of the clinical skills centre.

REASONS FOR SIMULATION

Teachers should be familiar with the role that simulation can play in a training programme. There are many reasons why simulation is seen as an essential rather than an optional element:

- 'Real patients' may not always be available for clinical teaching. With changes in healthcare delivery patients' stay in hospital is now shorter and during their stay they are occupied with investigation and treatment procedures. Patients may be less willing to have repeated exposure to students.
- With simulation every student can receive a guaranteed and standard clinical experience. Unlike with real patients a simulated experience can be made available to students at the most appropriate time to fit in with their learning programme.
- Repetitive practice is recognised as a key element in the acquisition of clinical skills. Learners can practise with the simulator until they have achieved the necessary mastery of the skill.
- Students are now introduced to clinical experiences earlier in many curricula and preparation on simulated patients and simulators can prepare them for their work with real patients.
- Trainees can be exposed to uncommon situations or rare clinical events that they may not encounter in their routine clinical experience.

- The management of crisis events can be practised and rehearsed so that students and trainees are better prepared should such events occur in real life. Airline pilots are trained in this way and simulators enable the pilots to deal with extreme situations such as engine failures.
- Students can learn a procedure in a risk-free environment. Learners can make mistakes and appreciate their consequences without causing harm to patients. Indeed in some areas it is now a requirement that a doctor demonstrates mastery of a procedure on a simulator before being approved to perform it on a patient. Uncoupling injury from learning sends a message to the public that patients are not 'a commodity' for training.
- Doctors need to be able to work as a member of a team. Simulation can address not only the acquisition of individual technical skills but also be used to train the learner to work in a coordinated and effective manner as a member of a team.
- The assessment of a learner's mastery of a clinical skill is important. Simulated patients and simulators can be used for this purpose in examinations, including high stakes examinations, to assess the learner's mastery of a skill as described in Section 5.
- Simulation can be used to provide students with a motivating and engaging learning experience. This can be designed to challenge the students, encourage their reflection and provide feedback about their performance. The experience can be customised to meet the needs of the individual learner.

APPROACHES TO SIMULATION

There are three approaches to simulating the real patient:

1. *Simulated patients.* These are individuals trained to play the role of a patient.
2. *Simulators or manikins.* These are devices or models that represent the functioning of the body or part of the body and with which the student can interact.
3. *Virtual patients.* The patient is represented in a computer simulation.

A hybrid approach has been developed by Kneebone and others that skilfully combines different patient simulations. A simulated patient, for example, can be used with a pelvic model attached. The student catheterises the 'patient', while at the same time communicating about the procedure with the simulated patient.

CHOICE OF SIMULATION

A number of factors should be taken into consideration when choosing the simulation approach to be adopted:

- **The expected learning outcomes.** Simulated patients are the obvious choice if communication skills are the expected learning outcome. Computer-based programs designed for the purpose also have a role to play in communication skills training. If skills in auscultation are the required learning outcome, a manikin such as the Harvey cardiac simulator is appropriate. Virtual patients can contribute to decision-making, problem-solving and patient-management skills.

- **The level of fidelity required.** Simulators vary in how similar they are to the real situation they are designed to simulate. A high fidelity simulator may be unnecessarily complex and expensive, and a simple piece of plastic simulating a wound on the skin may be adequate to teach suturing skills. A higher fidelity simulator may be required in a high stakes examination but may not always be necessary in a training situation. However, students tend to be more engaged with a high fidelity simulation that more closely resembles a patient.
- **The availability of simulators.** This may be a limiting factor. If students do not have immediate access to a clinical skills centre with a full range of simulators, it may be possible to arrange access to a nearby centre. If a bank of simulated patients is not available, a simulated patient can be trained to meet the needs of a programme but this can be time consuming. Virtual patients that can be shared online across institutions and modified to suit a local context are now available.

SIMULATED PATIENTS

A simulated patient is a person who has undergone various levels of training to portray a role or mimic a particular physical sign for the purposes of teaching or assessment. The term 'standardised patient' has been used when the person has been trained to play the role of a patient consistently and according to specific criteria. There are circumstances where a high degree of reproducibility is required in order that each student faces the same situation. This is important in the context of assessment.

Students interact with simulated patients as though they were taking a history from a real patient or examining or counselling them. Uses of simulated patients include:

- teaching and assessing history-taking and communication skills
- providing the student with the experience of counselling a patient in a difficult or sensitive area such as cancer where the use of a real patient would be inappropriate
- teaching and assessing physical examination
- teaching and assessing intimate examination of the genitalia.

Barrows (1993) and others have described how simulated patients can mimic a wide range of physical findings from an acute abdomen to spasticity. Simulated patients can be trained to portray various levels of difficulty appropriate to the stage of the learner. The simulated patient may provide a simple account of his or her history on being questioned by the learner or the patient can be programmed to be aggressive and difficult with a confusing or muddled history. Simulated patients can be trained to represent different settings of care including ambulatory care and general practice. A special group of simulated patients are recruited specifically to provide students with opportunities to learn the skills of male and female genital and digital rectal examination and female breast examination.

A significant advantage of simulated patients is that the patient can be trained to provide the students with feedback about their performance.

RECRUITING AND TRAINING SIMULATED PATIENTS

Simulated patients may be professionally trained actors, lay volunteers or healthcare professionals. The training of simulated patients takes time and effort and with a new recruit it is estimated that about two to three hours is required to deliver a good simulation. More detailed training may be necessary if the simulation is complex or if the simulated patient is required to assess the student's performance and provide feedback. Some Clinical Skills Units develop and maintain a bank of simulated patients.

Real patients may be trained to present their history and findings for the purpose of teaching and assessment in the same way as simulated patients.

SIMULATORS (MANIKINS AND MODELS)

Over the last two decades, manikins or models have been increasingly used to simulate 'real' patients in the teaching of clinical and practical skills and are now part of mainstream medical education. Simulators enable learners to practise patient care in a controlled and safe environment. The level of the sophistication of the manikins and models varies. At one end of the spectrum, simple models can be used that allow students to practise their skills in breast examination, prostate examination, wound closure, catheterisation, injection techniques and many other techniques and procedures. At the other end of the spectrum there are sophisticated models such as 'Harvey' – a life-sized cardiovascular patient simulator that can depict the auscultatory, tactile and visual findings for a broad range of cardiac problems (Fig. 25.1).

Computers can be integrated into whole- or part-body manikins, controlling the model's physiology and with the output shown as graphic displays on a monitor. A further development is the use of computer-based haptic systems that provide the learners with tactile sensations.

Simulators vary in their sophistication with regard to the extent to which they mimic the real-life situation, whether they provide feedback to the learner and the range of tasks and abnormalities that can be simulated.

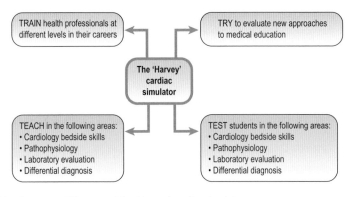

FIG 25.1 Examples of the uses of the 'Harvey' cardiac simulator.

There is good evidence that the skills gained from practice on a simulator transfer to real patients. Issenberg et al (2005) in a systematic review of the use of simulators identified key features that contribute to their educational effectiveness:

- **Provision of feedback.** Not surprisingly this was identified as an important feature of simulation-based medical education. (Feedback, the 'F' in 'FAIR', was discussed in Chapter 2.)
- **Repetitive practice.** Simulators provide an opportunity for learners to engage in *deliberate practice* where the learner engages in focused and repeated practice with the learning outcomes clearly defined. (Activity, the 'A' in 'FAIR'.)
- **Curriculum integration.** Simulation-based learning is most effective when it is embedded in the curriculum and not seen as some extraordinary event.
- **Range of difficulty level.** Effective learning is enhanced when learners have opportunities to engage in the practice of medical skills across a wide range of difficulty levels. (Individualisation, the 'I' in 'FAIR'.)
- **Capture of clinical variations.** The representation of a wide variety of problems or conditions as related to clinical practice. (Relevance, the 'R' in 'FAIR'.)
- **A non-threatening environment.** The use of simulators is most valuable where mistakes by learners are expected and not criticised, and where these are regarded as 'teachable moments'.
- **Individualised learning.** The learning on the simulator should be adapted to individual learning needs. This may mean that some students will require longer and more practice on the simulator than others. The level of difficulty of the presentation on the simulator may be altered to match the needs of the student. (Individualisation, the 'I' in 'FAIR'.)
- **Defined outcomes.** The expected learning outcomes for using the simulator should be defined and related to the overall outcomes of the curriculum. (Relevance, the 'R' in FAIR.)

COMPUTER SIMULATIONS AND VIRTUAL PATIENTS

Real patients can be simulated electronically as virtual patients that can be used in interactive computer simulations of real-life scenarios. The virtual patient has two components:

1. information about the patient including history, physical findings, laboratory and other investigations and the patient's progress
2. the learner's interaction with the case.

ADVANTAGES OF VIRTUAL PATIENTS

Virtual patients can be accessed on demand, perhaps even more so than simulated patients and manikin simulators, making them a very useful educational tool that offers a number of advantages:

- Virtual patients can be used to provide students with a wider range of patient scenarios than they may encounter in the real situation.
- The learner can take on the role of the doctor and no harm can result from any mistakes made.

- A holistic approach to patient management can be encouraged. The learner can interact with the patient and engage in reflection and clinical reasoning, while at the same time recognising professional and ethical issues.
- The virtual patient can highlight the integration of theory and practice, and the basic sciences with clinical medicine.
- Virtual patients can be used for teaching and learning and for assessing learners with the learners receiving feedback.
- Virtual patients can demonstrate the continuity of care with the same patient located over time in different contexts including general practice and the hospital setting.

USES OF VIRTUAL PATIENTS

Virtual patients can be used in a number of ways, for example:

- to support a traditional curriculum or learning programme, complementing the lecture and clinical experiences
- as the triggers or problem presentation in a problem-based learning curriculum (see Chapter 14)
- to support independent learning with students individually working through the case scenarios
- in collaborative learning with students working through a virtual patient scenario in pairs or in a group.

With technology developments, virtual patients are now more freely available on the internet or from commercial sources. In the past the wide range of instructional design and authoring tools had a negative impact on the transferability and sharing of virtual patients between different centres and institutions. Virtual patients developed in one context could not be adapted for use in another context and it was difficult if not impossible for teachers to alter a patient's presentation or investigations to fit in with their own context. There has been a significant move to more collaborative development and sharing of virtual patients with the implementation of a common standards specification. The Medbiquitous Virtual Patient standard has provided a stimulus.

As technology advances it is likely that we will see increasing use made of virtual patients in the training and assessment of students and trainees in all phases of their education.

CLINICAL SKILLS CENTRES

There has been a growing interest in the role of clinical skills centres as a setting for teaching and learning clinical skills. A clinical skills centre is usually a central area that houses a range of resources including simulators and simulated patients that can be used to assist students to master the appropriate clinical skills. The experiences students gain in a centre complement their dealings with real patients in other clinical contexts. Inter-professional education, with joint learning for different healthcare professionals, can successfully take place in the 'neutral setting' of such centres.

REFLECT AND REACT

1. Simulation is a powerful teaching and learning tool in medical education and a rich variety of simulators are now available. Some of these may be readily available to your students or trainees while others including high fidelity manikins may only be available in a central facility such as a clinical skills unit. What simulators do your students have access to?
2. Could greater use be made in your training programme of simulators, simulated patients or virtual patients? Which of the reasons given for simulation apply in your situation?
3. Prepare students for their simulated experience. This includes briefing the students about the expected learning outcomes and what is expected of them in the session. You should familiarise yourself with the simulation prior to the teaching session.
4. Work with the students during their use of the simulator. The extent to which you do this will vary depending on the complexity of the simulator and what is expected of the students.
5. Debrief the students following the simulation. This is an essential part of the process and will allow you to review what the students have learned and to provide them with feedback.

EXPLORING FURTHER

IF YOU HAVE A FEW HOURS

Barrows, H.S., 1993. An overview of the uses of standardized patients for teaching and evaluating clinical skills. Acad. Med. 68, 443–453.
An early account of how simulated patients can be used in medical education.

Berman, N.B., Fall, L.H., Chessman, A.W., et al., 2011. A collaborative model for developing and maintaining virtual patients for medical education. Med. Teach. 33, 319–324.
A description of how virtual patients can be shared between centres.

Cleland, J.A., Abe, K., Rethans, J.J., 2009. The use of simulated patients in medical education. AMEE Guide No. 42 Med. Teach. 31, 477–486.
A useful practical guide.

Collins, J.P., Harden, R.M., 1998. The use of real patients, simulated patients and simulators in clinical examinations. AMEE Guide No. 13 Med. Teach. 20, 508–521.
A description of how patients can be represented for teaching and assessment purposes.

Huang, G., Reynolds, R., Candler, C., 2007. Virtual patient simulation at U.S. and Canadian medical schools. Acad. Med. 82, 446–451.
An exploration of the educational value of virtual patients.

Issenberg, S.B., McGaghie, W.C., Petrusa, E.R., et al., 2005. Features and uses of high-fidelity medical simulations that lead to effective learning. BEME Guide No. 4. Med. Teach. 27, 10–28.
A review of the use of simulators and a description of the features that can lead to effective learning.

Med. Teach. 2009. 31 (8), 683–770.
This issue of Medical Teacher has virtual patients as its theme.

E-learning

The internet and resources available online have revolutionised medical education. They can make a significant contribution to your education programme.

INTRODUCTION

Lectures, small group teaching, teaching in the clinical context and independent learning all have an important role to play in an educational programme as described earlier in this section. E-learning too is now considered mainstream medical education. It is no longer a fad for the technologist or computer enthusiast, or an esoteric application used by a few innovators in the field. It has become part of and integrated into most educational programmes.

E-learning has been shown to be capable of making a difference with regard to the students' learning. Almost every student in a medical school and every trainee doctor spends part of his or her day or week online. They search for information on a topic using Google or some other search engine, communicate with a colleague or teacher, or study a unit, module or course developed in their institution or elsewhere.

WHAT IS E-LEARNING?

E-learning refers to 'electronic learning', in which instruction is delivered through a wide range of electronic means including computer and internet enabled learning. E-learning is recognised as being more than just technology and includes the social dynamics of networking.

Examples of e-learning include:

- independent learning using learning modules available online
- access to information and learning resources online
- web-based synchronous presentation by a teacher to a group of students
- students learning together online in real time, facilitated by a tutor
- asynchronous discussion forums or chat rooms and bulletin boards
- social networks such as Facebook
- interactive multi-media activities including games and simulations online or on a DVD
- virtual patients with whom the learner has to interact
- videos or audio recordings of lectures distributed through online streaming and podcasts using mobile devices such as telephones.

REASONS FOR INTRODUCING E-LEARNING

E-learning encompasses a pedagogical approach that can serve as a response to the challenges and developments confronting medical education. These include:

- an emphasis on student-centred and individualised learning with 'just-for-you' learning, 'just-in-time' learning and 'just-the-right-place' learning
- distributed learning with students learning at different sites
- increased access to medical studies for students from different backgrounds with programmes required to cater for an increasingly diverse group of students
- advances in medicine with the problem of information overload
- the continuum of education from undergraduate through postgraduate to continuing medical education
- international dimensions and globalisation with an expansion of the traditional classroom to include students from around the world
- the changing roles of a doctor with the need to learn new skills and acquire new competencies at different times in their career
- acquisition of the skills and tools that learners need to develop in order to prosper in an information society
- high expectations of students – the 'digital natives' – who come to medical school with more than 10 000 hours experience in e-learning
- collaborative or peer-to-peer learning, which can be significantly facilitated by social media networking
- inter-professional education with non-threatening learning opportunities online where doctors, nurses and other members of the healthcare team can participate
- sharing of rich learning resources with potential financial benefits.

E-learning has an important contribution to make in all of these areas and can serve as the solution or be part of the solution to the challenges.

EDUCATIONAL FEATURES

E-learning can be designed to deliver more effectively and efficiently what can be done with more traditional approaches. Alternatively e-learning can help to bring about a paradigm shift in medical education and serve as a response to the challenges described above. It has been suggested that, like a Trojan horse, e-learning can be introduced not just for the attributes it brings with it but also for the hidden curricular changes included.

E-learning meets the criteria specified in the CRISIS framework for effective continuing education (Fig. 26.1):

Convenience: students and trainees can learn anytime and anywhere.
Relevance: theory can be related to practice with on-the-job learning and the use of virtual patients extending the learner's clinical experience.
Individualisation: e-learning can be designed to meet the needs of individual students in terms of their past experience and learning styles.
Self-assessment: students can be assisted to assess their own competence through questions and assessment opportunities incorporated into the e-learning activity.

Interest: e-learning can be dynamic, engaging, and user friendly if properly developed.
Systematic: an e-learning programme can systematically cover a topic and a curriculum map can be embodied that provides a framework for the student's learning.

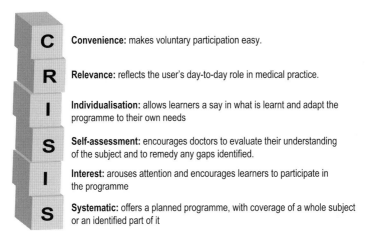

C Convenience: makes voluntary participation easy.

R Relevance: reflects the user's day-to-day role in medical practice.

I Individualisation: allows learners a say in what is learnt and adapt the programme to their own needs

S Self-assessment: encourages doctors to evaluate their understanding of the subject and to remedy any gaps identified.

I Interest: arouses attention and encourages learners to participate in the programme

S Systematic: offers a planned programme, with coverage of a whole subject or an identified part of it

FIG 26.1 The CRISIS framework for effective learning.

THE ROLE OF THE TEACHER

In e-learning the teacher is not redundant. Good collaboration is necessary between content experts, educationists and technologists. All of the roles for the teacher described in Chapter 1 are required but the emphasis in e-learning differs to some extent from what is expected in more traditional situations.

INFORMATION PROVIDER

Information normally provided in a lecture can be made more readily accessible to students through online downloads and podcasts. Existing lectures can be recorded or preferably reformatted to include a greater level of student interaction. The aim is to present information in a way that engages the learner, encourages interaction and tailors the learning to the needs of individual students. Video clips of experts presenting a topic or demonstrating a procedure can be made available to be used at a time most suitable for the learner.

Students worldwide can join live synchronous presentations by a lecturer using web-based platforms such as Wimba.

The role of the teacher is not simply to provide the student with information. The teacher's responsibility is to provide for the student the key to open the door to the rapidly expanding amount of available information. Students should be given guidance on the use of tools such as Wikipedia, YouTube and Google.

ROLE MODEL

Teachers facilitating learning online serve as role models for the students and can play an important part in shaping their attitudes and professionalism. Unfortunately staff may not be the best role models with regard to the use of e-learning or how information is accessed online. Prensky (2006) has described students as the 'digital natives' and staff as the 'digital immigrants'.

FACILITATOR

In e-learning the role of the teacher shifts significantly from delivering information and knowledge to one of supporting the learner. This can be done in a number of ways. Teachers can encourage and help students to acquire the skills of finding out information for themselves, and can guide the students with regard to accessing and assessing the quality of sources of information. In online collaborative learning the teacher has an important role as an e-tutor or e-mentor. Working with learners online requires particular competencies and approaches by the tutor.

ASSESSOR

Computers and information technology have an important role to play in assessment by making it possible for an assessment component to be incorporated into learning resources. Students can be encouraged to assess their achievement of the learning outcomes and to adjust if necessary their pace and path through the learning programme. Assessment should be viewed no longer as 'assessment *of* learning' but 'assessment *for* learning' and this provides a richer learning experience for the student. This concept is highlighted in Chapter 28.

Computers can be used to improve the effectiveness and efficiency of delivering traditional examinations, in scoring the student responses, and in the provision of feedback to the learner. Progress has been made with regard to online assessment for both formative and summative purposes. While the approach offers potential benefits it needs to be carefully managed to ensure that the examination runs smoothly. With summative assessment it is essential to ensure that adequate hardware and back-up systems are available. The AMEE Guide 39 covers many of the issues of online e-assessment (Dennick et al 2009).

The future may see the development of new approaches to assessment including adaptive assessment based on individual student responses and more authentic assessment related to medical practice.

CURRICULUM PLANNER

It is unusual to find in medicine a course that is entirely based on e-learning. There is a growing trend for a blended learning environment where the best of e-learning is combined with the best of face-to-face instruction. We are seeing a convergence between two learning environments and this may be the single greatest unrecognised trend in higher education today. The challenge for the teacher or trainer is to plan a curriculum that embraces both approaches.

Planning a blended approach may mean reconceptualising the role of lectures and placing a greater emphasis on independent learning. It gives the teacher the opportunity to provide students with learning experiences that might not otherwise be accessible to them and to offer a more student-centred approach to learning. The curriculum can be planned round a virtual practice. It can provide more personalised adaptive learning geared to the students' individual needs and opportunities can be scheduled for collaborative learning with students working together locally and internationally. In a problem-based learning discussion group, the problem may be presented to the student as an online simulation. When the need for further information is identified during the discussions, students can search for this online.

Some medical schools and some postgraduate bodies have made an organisational commitment to blend face-to-face and computer-based learning while others have ignored the opportunities offered. In one school we visited, e-learning had been rejected by the teachers with no e-learning contribution scheduled in the formal curriculum. We found on talking with the students that they were making their own arrangements and on average were spending 2½ hours a day online networking, emailing, or studying material they had personally found on the web.

With time, e-learning will feature more prominently in the medical curriculum and should not be ignored by curriculum planners or course designers.

RESOURCE DEVELOPER

The development of resources that combine appropriately the pedagogy and the technology is not an easy task. It requires a range of specialised skills that few teachers possess. A team approach is necessary involving content expert, instructional designer, educationist and technologist. Much has been written about this subject, and the 10 steps in the production of an e-learning programme are described in an AMEE guide (Harden et al 2012).

Most teachers will not wish or have the time to engage in the development from scratch of an e-learning programme. There are simpler ways to make a contribution. Resources can be created in the form of podcasts or recorded lectures. While this approach has limitations, in practice it has been found to serve a useful purpose. Another option is for teachers to use material that has already been developed and, if copyright permits, incorporate all or part of it into their own teaching programme. An animated sequence or a simulated patient can be incorporated into a lecture or self-learning programme. Repositories such as MedEd Portal offer a variety of content including video clips, images and self-assessment exercises.

If learning resources are identified as being of possible use for students, value can be added if the content is annotated by the teacher in order to put it in the perspective of the local context. Information about the resources with the annotations can be incorporated into the student's study guide.

If teachers are more ambitious, and with the author's permission, the published material can be used as a starting point to build their own resources. A number of authoring systems are available that can help teachers who lack the necessary technical expertise to create their own e-learning programme.

E-learning

REFLECT AND REACT

1. The future is blended learning. As a teacher think what this means for you in your course and whether you have the optimum mix of face-to-face and e-learning.
2. Be aware of the range of tools available including synchronous and asynchronous online learning, podcasts and social media.
3. Consider your role in e-learning. Do you serve as a role model for your students with regard to accessing information online and using learning resources?
4. Is your aim to make your teaching more effective and efficient using e-learning or is your aim to use e-learning to benefit your students in ways not otherwise possible, for example by personalising their learning?

EXPLORING FURTHER

IF YOU HAVE A FEW HOURS

Cartwright, C.A., Korsen, N., Urbach, L.E., 2002. Teaching the teachers: helping faculty in a family practice residency improve their informatics skills. Acad. Med. 77, 385–391.
This article describes how teachers can become role models for their students in the area of informatics.

Dennick, R., Wilkinson, S., Purcell, N., 2009. Online eAssessment. AMEE Guide No. 39. Med. Teach. 31, 192–206.

Ellaway, R., Masters, K., 2008. e-Learning in Medical Education. AMEE Guide No. 32. AMEE, Dundee.
A description of how e-learning is now part of mainstream medical education.

Harden, et al., 2012. Ten steps in planning an e-learning course. AMEE Guide. In press.
A practical guide to the production of an e-learning programme.

Med. Teach. 2011. 33 (4), 265–333.
This themed issue includes a number of articles on the current situation and future development with regard to e-learning.

McKendree, J., 2010. E-learning. In: Swanwick, T. (Ed.), Understanding Medical Education: Evidence, Theory and Practice. Wiley-Blackwell, Chichester, pp. 151–163 (Chapter 11).
Effective e-learning should be viewed as a curriculum design issue.

Ruiz, J.G., Mintzer, M.J., Leipzig, R.M., 2006. The impact of e-learning in medical education. Acad. Med. 81, 207–212.
A comprehensive introduction to e-learning.

Sandars, J.E., 2011. M-learning. In: Dent, J., Harden, R.M. (Eds.), A Practical Guide for Medical Teachers. Elsevier, London (Chapter 32).
A description of how mobile devices can be used to create new possibilities for teaching and learning on the move.

IF YOU HAVE MORE TIME

Clark, R.C., Mayer, R.E., 2007. E-learning and the Science of Instruction – Proven Guidelines for Consumers and Designers of Multimedia Learning, second ed. Jossey Bass, Chichester.
An introduction to some of the theory underpinning the use of e-learning.

Littlejohn, A., Pegler, C., 2007. Preparing for Blended E-learning. Routledge, London.
A description of the core skills required by teachers in blended learning.

Prensky, M., 2006. In: Don't Bother Me Mom – I'm Learning! How Computer and Video Games Are Preparing Your Kids For Twenty-first Century Success – and How You Can Help! Paragon House, Minnesota (Chapter 4).

Peer and collaborative learning

Students learning from each other is effective. This can be informal or incorporated into scheduled activities.

INTRODUCTION

Watching my 5-year-old grandson learn to use a computer, I (RMH) noted that he did not learn from the instruction manual, from his parents or from instruction at school. He learned from his 7-year-old sister. This is not surprising. Much of what we learn in day-to-day life is from friends and colleagues. It has always been a feature of how students learn at medical school. The difference today is that the value of learning in this way is appreciated and is given a more formal role in the curriculum. Students engaged in peer-to-peer (P2P) and collaborative learning tend to have a greater mastery of the expected learning outcomes with higher test scores, higher self-esteem, greater interpersonal skills and a greater understanding of the content they are studying.

DEFINITION

A range of terms such as 'P2P learning', 'collaborative learning' and 'cooperative learning' have been used to describe how students can learn with and from each other in formal and informal settings. Distinctions are sometimes drawn between the terms but frequently they are used interchangeably.

P2P LEARNING

P2P learning has been defined by Topping (1996) as 'people from similar social groupings who are not professional teachers helping each other to learn and learning themselves by teaching'. One student assumes the role of teacher or tutor while other students assume the role of learners or tutees. Students may switch their role from tutor to tutee. Usually, to guide students in their role as tutor, some instruction is given in teaching skills.

COLLABORATIVE LEARNING

In collaborative learning students learn from each other without the assignment of specific roles of tutor and tutee. Students work together as members of a group or team to solve a problem, complete a task or create a product. It is through working together that students learn. There is a sharing of authority and acceptance of responsibility among group members for the group's actions. The group may be assessed by the activity and product of the group rather than the individual's activity or achievements within the group. The term 'cooperative learning' rather than 'collaborative learning' has been used where there is more structure and organisation given to the group activity but the terms are often used interchangeably.

EXAMPLES OF P2P AND COLLABORATIVE LEARNING

P2P or collaborative learning may be adopted in the medical curriculum in a range of formats (we have not distinguished between the two approaches as there is often an overlap):

- Students are given the role of tutor in slots scheduled in the curriculum.
- Students form informal partnerships to assist each other.
- Students work in groups in the context of problem- or team-based learning.
- Students work in pairs facilitating each other's learning.
- Students collaborate in a project or in practical work such as anatomical dissection.
- Students work as members of an inter-professional group in a community-based project.
- Students work online as members of a formal discussion group with a specific task as the focus.
- Students share their experiences and information with others through a social network such as Facebook.
- Students collaborate in the development of educational resources or textbooks that they share with others.
- Students have the responsibility for assessing each other's achievements in an area such as professionalism (peer assessment).
- Students in more senior years or junior doctors teach junior students.

BENEFITS TO BE GAINED BY P2P AND COLLABORATIVE LEARNING

The institution or medical school and the learner can benefit in a number of ways if collaborative learning is incorporated in the curriculum:

- Students can learn effectively from their peers, in particular where there are problems relating to complex learning and concept manipulation.
- Learning outcomes less easily achieved through other methods are promoted. These include interpersonal skills, communication skills, higher level thinking skills, skills of critical appraisal and team working skills.
- Students are helped to develop their confidence and self esteem.
- Students are prepared for life-long learning as the classroom more closely resembles real-life social and employment situations.
- Students' satisfaction with the learning experience is enhanced with a more positive attitude developed towards the subject matter.

- Students are encouraged to appreciate diversity and to reflect and appreciate different viewpoints and perspectives brought to the discussion by other students.
- Learners working online at a distance have a supportive community environment.
- Additional support for student learning is provided at a time when there is pressure on staff:student ratios.
- An educational environment is created within the institution where collaboration is valued.
- A student-centred learning approach is supported with students taking more responsibility for their own learning.
- Teaching is a powerful learning tool – 'to teach is to learn twice'.
- Students' skills as teachers are developed in line with recommendations from accrediting bodies that medical graduates must be able to demonstrate appropriate teaching skills.
- Students feel engaged and have some ownership of the curriculum.
- The concept of the student as an assessor of other students is supported, in particular in areas such as attitudes and professionalism.
- Students receive significant feedback as part of the learning activity which is not always possible in other situations, particularly in large group learning.
- Experience gained as a student teacher may encourage some students to seek an academic career.

IMPLEMENTATION IN PRACTICE

The successful implementation of P2P and collaborative learning has much in common with the general curriculum development principles described elsewhere in this book. It is important to clarify the expected learning outcomes, to ensure that planning and preparation is adequate, that the process is facilitated by an appropriate education environment, and that there is a match between assessment and teaching and learning. Some specific recommendations are noted below.

P2P LEARNING

The following tips contribute to successful P2P learning:

- Incorporate P2P learning formally into the curriculum and do not consider it only as an add-on extra.
- Schedule the P2P sessions and make the necessary arrangements for students to sign up.
- Decide whether students' attendance is obligatory or whether the P2P sessions are optional.
- Ensure that both the tutors and tutees are aware of how P2P learning contributes to the mastery of the learning outcomes of the course. It is sometimes claimed that the tutor gains as much if not more than the tutee. This includes mastery of teaching skills.
- Ensure that student tutors are fully briefed and have training in the necessary skills. They may be assisted with the provision of learning resources to support the learning.

- P2P tutors should have ongoing mentoring and coaching by staff.
- Choose the form of P2P learning that is most appropriate for your situation. This may involve students in the same year or more senior students or junior doctors acting as tutors.
- In planning and organising P2P learning, a team approach involving both staff and students is useful.
- As with all learning experiences P2P learning should be monitored and evaluated.

COLLABORATIVE LEARNING

The success of collaborative learning can depend on how it is implemented:

- Explain to the students the benefits of the collaborative learning approach and the expected learning outcomes, including the development of interpersonal skills and mastery of the subject content. It is important that they accept them.
- Collaborative learning can be at its most effective with heterogeneous groups where students tend to interact and achieve more compared to working with students more closely matched in their abilities and background.
- The learning tasks can be structured so that students must depend on each other for completion of the task. This involves within the group trust building, conflict management, encouragement and negotiation. Each student should be held accountable for doing their own share of the work. One inter-professional group we saw, as described in Chapter 13, worked well because the solution to the problem presented required the theoretical knowledge of the medical student members of the group and the practical knowledge of the midwives.
- It is important that sufficient time is allocated to collaborative learning. Students need to complete the required tasks and achieve the expected learning outcomes. This creates an atmosphere of achievement in the group. Some of the social benefits may become apparent only after the group has worked together for a number of weeks.
- Students should have the opportunity within their small group to reflect upon and reply to the diverse responses from other group members. The exchange of views in the group should help students to understand better the issues and concepts being discussed.
- It is important to recognise that just because students are working in small groups it does not mean that they are engaging in collaborative learning. It needs to be ensured that students are cooperating with regard to their own learning and the learning of others in the group.
- Each member of the group should contribute to the work and product of the group so that the end result will be better than that achieved by one student, even the best, working independently.
- Encourage students in the group to explain concepts or principles to others and for the explanation to be discussed by the group. This can lead to effective learning for the members of the group.

- The group activities should be organised in such a way that the learning success of each individual and the group as a whole is recognised. We saw this achieved in one setting where an individual was chosen by the teacher at random at the end of the week to present the work of the group. The group was given a mark based on the individual's presentation. The group had to 'sink or swim' together.
- Monitor the group activity and the progress being made by the students in the group. The teacher, when facilitating a group should provide assistance and clarification if required. It is important that the teacher does not dominate the session and convert it into a mini-lecture.

REFLECT AND REACT

1. You may feel uncomfortable delegating teaching responsibilities to a student or trainee. There is overwhelming evidence that this can be effective. Consider how it can be adopted in your situation.
2. Which of the advantages of P2P or collaborative learning listed above apply in your situation?
3. Look at the learning outcomes for your course or curriculum and consider whether some outcomes such as team work could be usefully addressed through P2P or collaborative learning.

EXPLORING FURTHER

IF YOU HAVE A FEW HOURS

Ross, M.T., Cameron, H.S., 2007. Peer assisted learning: a planning and implementation framework. AMEE Guide No. 30. Med. Teach. 29, 527–545.
A description of how P2P learning can be implemented based on experience at Edinburgh Medical School.

Topping, K.J., 1996. The effectiveness of peer tutoring in further and higher education: A typology and review of the literature. High. Educ. 32, 321–345.
A report from an expert in the field.

IF YOU HAVE MORE TIME

Boud, D., Cohen, R., Sampson, J. (Eds.), 2001. Peer Learning in Higher Education: Learning from and with Each Other. Kogan Page, London.

McConnell, D., 2006. E-Learning Groups and Communities. The Society for Research into Higher Education and Open University Press, Maidenhead.

SECTION 5
ASSESSING THE PROGRESS OF THE LEARNER

'Lack of assessment and feedback, based on observation of performance in the workplace, is one of the most serious deficiencies in current medical education practice.'
John Norcini and Vanessa Burch 2007

OVERVIEW

The assessing of the learner is arguably the most important task for the teacher. Students can walk away from bad teaching, but they cannot avoid bad assessment.

Chapter 28 Six questions to ask about assessment
An understanding of basic concepts and approaches will help you to do a good job.

Chapter 29 Written and computer-based assessment
Written questions have a role to play alongside other assessment methods.

Chapter 30 Clinical and performance-based assessment
An assessment of a student's clinical competence is key to an assessment of their ability to practise medicine.

Chapter 31 Portfolio assessment
Portfolio assessment is a response to changes in medical education including the emphasis on professionalism and the need to give students more responsibility for their own learning.

Chapter 32 Assessment for admission to medicine and postgraduate training
A range of assessment tools and approaches are available to assist with key selection decisions.

Chapter 33 Evaluating the curriculum
Curriculum evaluation is an essential part of the educational process. The focus in curriculum evaluation is on quality improvement.

Six questions to ask about assessment

An understanding of basic concepts and approaches will help you to do a good job.

The assessment of a student's or trainee's learning is important not only for the student or trainee but also for the teacher, the course organiser, the accrediting body and the public as the consumer. Important decisions are taken about students as a result of the scores they achieve in examinations. Teachers and the other stakeholders need to know if students have achieved the appropriate level of mastery to move on to the next part of their training programme and if, on completion of their training, they are competent to practise as a doctor in a particular context.

Although assessment is important, it is one of the most difficult areas in medical education on which to get agreement. What constitutes a fair examination and what are the criteria for passing a student? Assessment is an area in which there have been significant developments as to what constitutes 'good practice' and these will be highlighted in this chapter.

Assessment procedures have been criticised by students, by professional bodies and by those outside medicine. In a recent court case, a judge criticised a nursing school for a failure to identify in its assessment procedures a nurse who proved grossly incompetent and demonstrated unprofessional behaviour after she qualified. For the student, assessment may be seen as analogous to playing in a cricket match where the rules have not been clearly specified in advance and are constantly being changed by the umpire. Students may perceive the examiner as threatening and as someone whose aim is to catch them out and find fault with them (Figs 28.1 and 28.2).

Problems with assessment are serious: students can walk away from bad teaching but they are unable to do so with assessment if they are to achieve the qualification they seek. That assessment is a key and integral part of curriculum development is often not recognised. Issues relating to assessment should be seen not only as a testing or measurement problem but as inextricably linked to the learning outcomes and teaching methods. Course design and assessment are inseparable.

When thinking about assessment it is useful to think about six questions:

1. Who should assess the student?
2. Why assess the student?
3. What should be assessed?

ASSESSING THE PROGRESS OF THE LEARNER

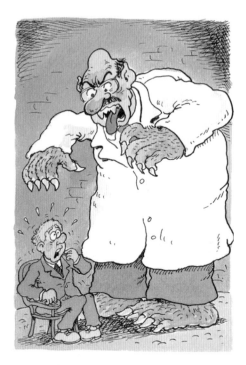

FIG 28.1 Students may perceive the examiner as threatening.

4. How should the student be assessed?
5. When should the student be assessed?
6. Where should the student be assessed?

It is important to think about the overall programme of assessment, including the tools used and how they are implemented, and not to overemphasise one aspect such as the psychometric properties of the assessment instruments.

WHO SHOULD ASSESS THE STUDENT?

One reason why assessment is complex and the teacher's responsibilities may be unclear is that there is a range of stakeholders involved. These include:

- international accrediting bodies
- national accrediting bodies such as the General Medical Council in the UK and, in the USA, The National Board of Medical Examiners
- professional bodies, for example the Royal Colleges in the UK and the National Boards in the USA
- the public and patients
- the individual school in which the student is enrolled
- the department or course committee responsible for teaching the subject
- the individual teacher
- the students themselves.

In medical schools in the UK, the assessment process is overseen by the General Medical Council (GMC) and the implementation is the responsibility

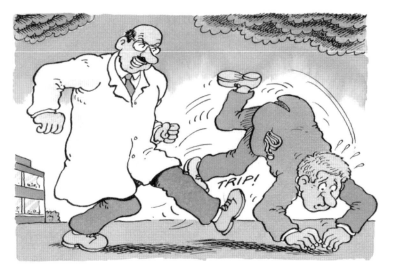

FIG 28.2 Students may perceive the examiner as someone whose aim is to catch them out.

of each medical school. Teachers from other schools serve as external examiners and participate in the development of the school's examinations, their implementation and pass/fail decisions. In contrast, in North America and in some other countries there is a national examination which students are required to pass. Each approach has merits. A national examination, while setting national standards, may stifle innovation in individual medical schools (Harden 2009).

In medical practice, doctors have to take responsibility for assessing their own performance and keeping themselves up-to-date. Not all doctors have the necessary skills or recognise the importance of the responsibility. Students must be prepared for this as part of their undergraduate education with reinforcement throughout their postgraduate training. Problems with unreliability in self-assessment are well recognised and there may also be problems with how students react to the assessment of their own competence. On one occasion, we asked students to mark their own examination paper against a model answer. Some found the procedure so traumatic that they were unable to complete the process and to our surprise required counselling as a result. Training students to become doctors who are inquirers into their own competence, and who are comfortable with this, should be a learning outcome of the curriculum.

Increasing attention is being paid to peer assessment, and the evaluation of students by their peers against certain learning outcomes has become part of some institutions' assessment strategy. This is particularly valuable in the assessment of attitudes where often the student body has a better understanding of individual students' strengths and weaknesses than the teachers.

WHY ASSESS THE STUDENT?

At an early stage in planning an assessment programme it is important to consider the purpose of the assessment. An assessment designed to certify a student's competence to practise as a trainee doctor will be different from the assessment method used to review a student's progress and provide feedback during course work. Traditionally, assessment has been described as either 'formative', where the main aim is to provide the learners with feedback about their progress, or 'summative' where the aim is to determine whether the learners have achieved the course objectives. This distinction has become blurred with the recognition that summative assessment can also be used to provide feedback to the learner and summative decisions may be based on evidence collected during the training programme.

The purposes that can be served by assessment include:

- **Decisions as to whether the learner is 'fit for purpose'.** Has the learner satisfactorily completed the training programme and achieved the standard expected by the public and professional bodies to practise as a trainee or as a specialist in a particular field of medicine?
- **Assessment of the student's progress during the education or training programme.** It is important to identify deficiencies early in a training programme so that these can be remedied without waiting until a final examination when it will be too late to take the necessary action. This is particularly true with regard to the assessment of behaviour and attitudes.
- **Grading or ranking the student with the aim of identifying the 'best' students among those being assessed.** This 'norm-referenced' approach to assessment is applicable when candidates have to be selected for a limited number of posts, or students selected for admission to medicine where only a set number of places are available. This approach to assessment should not be confused with a 'criterion-referenced' approach where the learner's achievement is assessed against the expected learning outcomes or a set of criteria.
- **Enhancing the student's learning.** Emphasis is placed on 'assessment for learning' rather than 'assessment of learning'. In addition to serving as a tool for accountability, assessment can be a tool to support and improve learning. This is consistent with an 'assessment-to-a-standard' approach where what matters are the standards students achieve rather than the time it takes them to do so.
- **Motivating the student.** It has been demonstrated that assessment has a powerful impact on students and is a major factor in driving their learning. In one medical school we found that, because there was no examination in the subject, students neglected otolaryngology despite the fact that the topic was taught in an imaginative problem-based way. When the subject was routinely included as a station in the final objective structured clinical examination (OSCE), the students' approach to studying the topic changed dramatically.
- **Provision of feedback for the teacher.** The teacher can glean useful information from the student assessment but all too often this source of information is untapped. The analysis of students' scores in one multiple choice question (MCQ) examination revealed that students had performed badly in a question relating to diabetes. This was subsequently found to be related to a weakness in the training programme which had to be addressed.

WHAT SHOULD BE ASSESSED?

A key feature of outcome-based education, as discussed in Section 2, is that assessment is matched closely with the specified learning outcomes. This is referred to as competency-based assessment. What we choose to assess in the education programme demonstrates what we value and many problems encountered with assessment arise from an inadequate consideration of what is being assessed. Assessment drives learning as we have described above. In the absence of a set of learning outcomes what is assessed becomes, for the students, the course objectives. In the past the emphasis in assessment was on the knowledge domain with less attention paid to skills and attitudes. There were a number of reasons for this. Mastery of knowledge was traditionally regarded as of greater importance than the development of attitudes. Knowledge was also easier to assess than other domains and there was a natural tendency to assess what was easy to assess and to shy away from areas where assessment was contentious or difficult. Written assessments, including MCQ papers which tested the knowledge domain, dominated assessment practice. However, someone who can answer correctly a set of MCQs is not necessarily a good doctor and there has been a move to assess in the student or doctor more complex achievement, higher order thinking, clinical skills, attitudes and professionalism.

The introduction of the OSCE stimulated the assessment of psychomotor and other performance related skills, and more recently the adoption of portfolio assessment and multi-source feedback has recognised the importance of the assessment of independent learning and self-assessment skills, attitudes and professionalism.

It is important that, with the many changes advocated in medical education and the different expectations we have of our students in today's curricula, assessment does not lag behind. What we assess must closely match what we expect students to learn.

HOW SHOULD THE STUDENT BE ASSESSED?

A wide range of tools or instruments are now available that can be used to assess the student's competence (Fig. 28.3). Some of these are described in the chapters that follow. Just as important as the assessment tool selected, if not more so, is the way in which the tool is employed. A good tool badly used will yield inappropriate or misleading results. We now have a better understanding of what makes a good assessment:

- **The method should be reliable and consistent.** This relates to the certainty with which a decision can be made about the student's performance on the basis of the test results. For a reliable assessment the measurement instrument must be relatively stable. It would not be good practice, for example, to use an elastic tape measure to measure length. The measurement would not be reliable.

  A factor that led to the widespread use of MCQs was that their high reliability could be demonstrated. Problems with reliability associated with tests of clinical competence were highlighted when we found that examiners watching the same clinical performance awarded different scores to the examinees

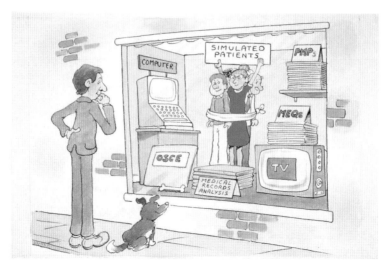

FIG 28.3 A range of assessment tools are available.

and, watching a video of the students' performance some weeks later, they were not consistent with the marks they had awarded. The problem of reliability was a factor which stimulated us to develop the OSCE.

- **The method should be valid.** In other words the assessment method should measure the learning outcomes intended (Fig. 28.4). The test should be an 'honest' one, testing what it purports to measure. There may be a trade-off at times between reliability and validity. This is illustrated in the classic story of the drunk man who was seen at night looking under a street light for his car keys which he had dropped. When asked why he was looking there when he had dropped them a short distance away, he replied that it was easier to see what was on the ground under the light. His search strategy, although having merit, was not valid in his situation.

  Reliability has been emphasised in the past at the expense of validity. What is needed is a test that is both valid and reliable. A test may be reliable but it is of no value if it does not measure what we want to measure. Unfortunately, the more simple a test, the more likely it is to be reliable while at the same time the less likely it is to be valid. Medicine by its nature

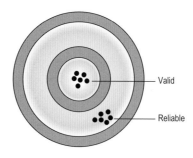

FIG 28.4 Tests should be valid as well as reliable.

is a complex subject and assessment of professionalism or communication skills is by necessity complex if it is to be valid.

- **The method should be feasible** in terms of the resources available and the number of students to be examined. The assessment scheme should not be overly complex and should be capable of being implemented by the teacher in routine practice.
- **The assessment should have a positive impact on the student's learning.** When we first introduced the OSCE in the final examination and included some stations with family physicians as examiners, we found that students spent less time in the library revising their theoretical knowledge and more time learning on the wards and in the community setting. This was in line with the aims of the curriculum.

STANDARD SETTING

A strategy should be adopted which serves as a basis for decisions as to whether a student has reached the standard required to pass the examination. A standard is a statement of whether a student's examination performance is good enough for a particular purpose. Relative or norm-referenced standards, as described above, are based on a comparison of a learner's performance with his or her peers: for example 75% of learners will pass. Absolute standards in contrast are based on the learner's performance in terms of set criteria: for example 60% of the MCQs answered will be correct. Much attention has been focused in recent years on methods of determining the standard expected of students in an examination. Should the pass mark be 60% or should it be 55% or 65% of questions answered correctly? Setting pass standards is a complex task and beyond the scope of this book. Useful introductions to setting standards in examinations can be found in the Exploring Further section at the end of the chapter.

WHEN SHOULD THE STUDENT BE ASSESSED?

Traditionally learners were assessed on their mastery of the subject in a set examination at the end of the course. Increasing emphasis has been placed on collecting evidence about the learner's achievement of the expected learning outcomes during their training or course of study. There are a number of reasons for this. Without the time constraints of a final examination, a much wider sample of the students' performance can be assessed, increasing the reliability of the examination. In addition, the assessment may be more valid in that the assessment tools that can be adopted during the course may assess learning outcomes difficult to assess in an end-of-course final examination. An important additional benefit of in-course assessment is that it provides feedback to the student and teacher and allows time for remediation.

Less frequently undertaken is the assessment of the student at the beginning of the training programme. A number of years ago, we asked third-year students at the beginning of their course in endocrinology to complete the end-of-course examination on day one of the course. The results were surprising. Some students scored less than 10% while other students scored almost

50%, the pass mark for the examination. This provided important evidence as to the need for a course in endocrinology which could be tailored to suit the abilities of the different students. Independent learning modules were developed which were used successfully to replace some lectures on the topic. It could be argued that our first student assessment is when we select students to enter medical studies, or select graduates for a postgraduate training programme (see Chapter 32).

WHERE SHOULD THE STUDENT BE ASSESSED?

Students have been assessed traditionally using written papers in an examination hall environment, or with formal clinical examinations in the hospital ward. With moves towards greater authenticity in assessment, and with assessment seen more as a continuous process, increased attention is being focused on assessment in the work place and in the wide range of contexts where teaching takes place, whether in the hospital or community environment. This is discussed further in Chapter 30.

REACT AND REFLECT

1. Assessment is frequently one of the last things considered when a curriculum is planned. It is often the first thing the learner thinks about. Have you spent enough time considering the assessment of learners in your programme?
2. From the list of purposes given above, what purposes are served by the examinations in your programme?
3. How would you rate your examination against the criteria given for a 'good assessment'?
4. What learning outcomes are assessed?

EXPLORING FURTHER

IF YOU HAVE A FEW HOURS

Bandaranayake, R.C., 2010. Setting and Maintaining Standards in Multiple Choice Examinations. AMEE Guide No. 37. AMEE, Dundee.
An account of the advantages and disadvantages of the more commonly used methods of setting standards in MCQ examinations.

Harden, R., 2009. Five myths and the case against a European or national licensing examination. Med. Teach. 31, 217–220.

Norcini, J., Anderson, B., Bollela, V., 2011. Criteria for good assessment: consensus statement and recommendations from the Ottawa 2010 conference. Med. Teach. 33, 206–214.
This article identifies the current issues in defining criteria for good assessment, makes recommendations on how to proceed and offers some guidance.

Norcini, J., McKinley, D.W., 2010. Standard setting. In: Dent, J.A., Harden, R.M. (Eds.), A Practical Guide for Medical Teachers. Elsevier, London (Chapter 41).
A review of some of the common methods for setting standards, and a framework for evaluating their credibility.

Shumway, J.M., Harden, R.M., 2003. AMEE Medical Education Guide No. 25. The assessment of learning outcomes for the competent and reflective physicians. Med. Teach. 25, 569–584.
A description of the assessment tools that can be used to assess the different outcome learning.

IF YOU HAVE MORE TIME

Downing, S.M., Yudkowsky, R. (Eds.), 2009. Assessment in Health Professions Education. Routledge, New York.
A comprehensive text devoted specifically to assessment in the health professions.

Gronlund, N.E., Waugh, C.K., 2009. Assessment of Student Achievement, ninth ed. Pearson Education, Upper Saddle River, New Jersey.
A classic text worthwhile consulting, particularly Chapter 1.

Hodges, B.D., Ginsburg, S., Cruess, R., et al., 2011. Assessment of professionalism: recommendations from the Ottawa 2010 conference. Med. Teach. 33, 354–363.
Different ways of thinking about professionalism that can lead toward a multi-dimensional, multi-paradigmatic approach to assessing professionalism at different levels: individual, inter-personal and societal-institutional.

Six questions to ask about assessment

Written and computer-based assessment

Written questions have a role to play alongside other assessment methods.

WRITTEN ASSESSMENT HAS A ROLE TO PLAY

Written approaches to assessment are well established and have been widely used to assess learners' competence in all spheres of education. Despite the greater emphasis being placed on performance assessment, written approaches still have an important role to play. The use of written examinations has come under scrutiny with regard to their match with the expected learning outcomes and their impact on the learners' behaviour. Alternative written assessment methods have been developed as a response to these challenges and increasingly computers have replaced paper and pencil techniques for the delivery of the assessment.

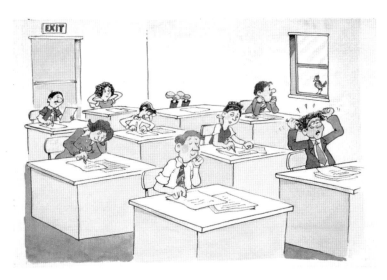

FIG 29.1   A written examination.

THE ELEMENTS IN WRITTEN ASSESSMENT

It is helpful to think of written assessment in terms of the stimulus or task that necessitates a learner's response, the response expected of the learner, the assessment of the student's response and the media or technology used.

THE STIMULUS

The stimulus for the learner's response may be:

- a short statement or question, e.g. 'In which of the following pathologies does a patient typically present with weight loss and an increased appetite?' or 'List the 3 options in the management of a patient with hyperthyroidism.'
- a statement or question with accompanying diagrams or charts, e.g. 'In the diagram which structure is labelled 'A'?'
- a short clinical scenario with a patient's presentation followed by a question, e.g. 'Mrs Wilkie, a 35-year-old waitress complaining of tiredness and nervousness...'
- a more extended patient management problem that develops over a period of time.

THE STUDENT'S RESPONSE

The response expected of the learner can be categorised into:

- Constructed response questions where the student has to write a long or short narrative in response to the stimulus. These include essays, short essay questions and short answer questions.
- Selected response questions where the student has to make a selection from a range of options provided. These include multiple choice questions (MCQs), for example the one best answer or multiple true/false questions and extended matching items.

THE ASSESSMENT OF THE STUDENT'S RESPONSE

The learner's response may be scored:

- Automatically correct or incorrect, as in an MCQ where there is an agreed correct answer. This also applies to short answer questions where the expected answer is limited to a few words. In this case, agreement has to be reached with regard to alternative wording and spelling that is acceptable.
- In a constructed response question, by an examiner based on a holistic impression of the student's response, or with an assigned structured marking scheme.
- In the context of the answers to the questions provided by members of a panel of experts. This is the strategy used in the script concordance test as described below.

STANDARD SETTING

The subject of standard setting was introduced in the previous chapter. A range of methods have been used in a written examination to determine the mark above which students will pass the examination and below which they will fail (Bandaranayake 2008).

It is not uncommon for a pass mark for an MCQ paper to be set at 60–70%. This implies, however, that students need to know only two thirds of the area covered and that it does not matter which third they do not know. Although it is not usual practice, consideration needs to be given to an examination or part of an examination that assesses essential core knowledge, with a pass mark of more than 90% expected for that part of the examination.

TYPES OF WRITTEN ASSESSMENT

ESSAY QUESTION

While the essay remains a common assessment tool in many fields, it is less commonly used in medicine. Provided the question or stimulus is appropriate, the essay can test:

- the learner's general understanding of the topic
- higher level skills including synthesis, organisation of information, analysis, problem solving and evaluation
- written communication skills, a competence often not tested by other written assessment methods although portfolio assessment may be used for this purpose
- aspects relating to attitudes and medical ethics.

Essay questions do have a number of disadvantages as an assessment tool:

- The content area sampled is small compared to an MCQ paper.
- The scoring of the questions is subjective and time consuming.

SHORT ESSAY QUESTION (SEQs)

Short essay questions are designed to sample a wider range of content than the essay question. A student may have to answer twelve 10-minute short essay questions instead of four 30-minute or two 1-hour essay questions. The SEQ has many of the advantages and disadvantages of the essay question.

SHORT ANSWER QUESTIONS (SAQs)

In a short answer question, rather than selecting from a list of choices as in a MCQ, the student is expected to respond to the question in one, two or a limited number of words. The format has the advantages of an MCQ in that a wide range of content can be sampled and has the added advantage that it does not simply test recognition of the correct answer from a list of options. It is also easier to set questions that test core or basic knowledge without having to cue the learner with the responses on a list. MCQs offer the advantage that they can be automatically marked but SAQs share this advantage and it is possible to mark an SAQ using the appropriate computer program, although agreement needs to be reached with regard to the answers that are acceptable. SAQs are now routinely used in examinations such as the progress test at the medical school in Dundee and merit wider consideration and adoption as an alternative to the MCQ.

MULTIPLE CHOICE QUESTIONS (MCQs)

Multiple choice questions can sample objectively a wide range of a student's knowledge and understanding. The downside for the examiner is not the marking of the responses but the setting of the questions. Several question banks have been developed in medicine and these allow schools to share questions.

Many MCQ examinations test mainly recall of knowledge rather than in-depth understanding or application. This has had a detrimental effect on how students study. To counteract this, there has been a move to introduce greater authenticity to the MCQ through the use of clinical scenarios in the stem or stimulus.

Many formats have been described but two approaches have dominated:

- Single best option where the learner is required to select the best response from four or five alternatives.
- Multiple true/false questions where the student has to categorise as true or false each of five statements relating to the stem. Guessing is a more important consideration with this type of question and as a result the marking scheme may be more complicated. There has been a move away from using this type of question although it does test a wider range of knowledge and the questions are easier to set without the need for distracters as in the single best option type of question.

EXTENDING MATCHING QUESTIONS (EMQs)

The EMQ is a type of written question in the selected response category that provides an alternative to the standard MCQ. The EMQ consists of a list of around 20 options relating to a theme or topic. This may be a list of drugs, diseases, laboratory investigations, symptoms, explanations or pathologies. Following the lead-in stem or stimulus, usually in the form of a patient scenario, the student has to select the most appropriate answer from the list of options. There may be one, two or more questions using the same list of options. An advantage is that, with the extended list of options from which the student has to select the answer, the effect of cuing as found in the MCQ is minimised. The questions are less time consuming to produce as several scenarios can use the same list of options. As with MCQs a computer can be used to score the answers.

MODIFIED ESSAY QUESTIONS (MEQs)

The MEQ is a sequence of questions based on a patient scenario that develops over a period of time. After the first question is answered, further information is provided about the patient and this is followed by another question. The typical MEQ may have six or more questions and both SAQs and MCQs may be used. There are difficulties with scoring this format and it is now rarely used.

SCRIPT CONCORDANCE TEST (SCT)

This is a relatively new form of written assessment. Students are given a brief patient scenario and asked to make judgements regarding diagnostic possibilities or management options. To allow decisions to be made that reflect medical practice, the student is given sufficient clinical detail but a certain amount of uncertainty, imprecision or incompleteness is deliberately built into each case in order to simulate real-life clinical situations. The scoring is based on the amount of agreement between the student and a panel of experts. The approach may be useful, particularly in the assessment of a student's clinical reasoning.

THE TECHNOLOGY

Questions can be posed, responses recorded and examinations scored either on paper or on a computer. Computers are now widely used for MCQs: the students answer on a computer and their responses are automatically scored. There is some interest in adaptive testing where the questions presented to the students on the computer are determined by their responses to earlier questions. A wrong answer to a question may generate additional related questions that allow the student's understanding or lack of understanding of the area to be explored further. This may increase the reliability of the examination by increasing the number of questions used in the areas where the student's understanding is in doubt. This approach is not in routine use at the moment.

REFLECT AND REACT

1. Given the learning outcomes to be tested and the resources available, which format of written test is appropriate to your setting?
2. To what extent does a written examination in your course test more than factual recall?
3. Consider how you can best provide feedback to students about their performance in a written examination. Simply providing a mark, for example 62%, is not sufficient.

EXPLORING FURTHER

IF YOU HAVE A FEW HOURS

Amin, Z., Boulet, J.R., Cook, D.A., et al., 2011. Technology-enabled assessment of health professions education: consensus statement and recommendations from the Ottawa 2010 Conference. Med. Teach. 33, 364–369.
This paper highlights the changing nature of ICT in assessment and the challenges that need to be addressed when technology is incorporated into assessment.

Bandaranayake, R.C., 2008. Setting and maintaining standards in multiple choice examinations. AMEE Guide No. 37. Med. Teach. 30, 836–845.
An account of the advantages and disadvantages of the more commonly used methods of setting standards in MCQ examinations.

Case, S.M., Swanson, D.B., 2002. Constructing Written Test Questions for the Basic and Clinical Sciences, third ed. (revised). National Board of Medical Examiners, Philadelphia.
A classic description of how to prepare MCQs.

IF YOU HAVE MORE TIME

Schuwirth, L.W.T., Van der Vleuten, C.P.M., 2010. Written assessment. In: Cantillon, P., Wood, D., (Eds.), ABC of Learning and Teaching in Medicine. second ed. (Chapter 9). John Wiley and Sons, Chichester.
A useful overview of the use of written examinations in medicine.

Clinical and performance-based assessment

30

An assessment of a student's clinical competence is key to an assessment of their ability to practise medicine.

THE IMPORTANCE OF CLINICAL ASSESSMENT

Written assessment instruments assess what students know and how they apply this knowledge to a written problem. Clinical and work-based assessment instruments assess the clinical and practical skills of the examinee and how knowledge is applied in the clinical context. The clinical examination is of key importance in the assessment of the learner's competence to practise medicine, and in many schools is the cornerstone in qualifying examinations.

The assessment of competence can be distinguished from performance assessment. Tests of competence, such as the objective structured clinical examination (OSCE), demonstrate in a controlled situation what an examinee is capable of doing. Performance assessment tools such as record analysis or multi-source feedback assess what the individual does in practice. The Miller pyramid provides a framework for assessment with the bottom of the pyramid being the assessment of knowledge and the higher levels of the pyramid being the assessment of performance (Fig. 30.1).

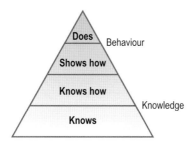

FIG 30.1 The Miller pyramid.

CONSIDERATIONS IN CLINICAL ASSESSMENT

THE PATIENT

Central to the clinical examination is the interaction of the examinee with a patient. The role of the patient in the encounter varies depending upon the type of interaction between the examinee and the patient expected. For the purpose of the examination, the patient may be a 'real' patient, a simulated patient or a computer representation used as a patient substitute.

There are benefits to be gained from the use of a range of patient representations in the clinical examination. The choice of patient representation will be influenced by what is being assessed, the level of standardisation required, the required realism or fidelity and the local logistics including the availability and relative costs associated with the use of real patients and trained simulated patients (Collins and Harden 1998).

'Real' patients

The traditional clinical examination was based on 'real' patients and they are the basis for the patient encounter in a work-based assessment. 'Real' patients are widely used in OSCE stations although this is less common in North America. The examination organisers may have access to a bank of patients with a range of pathologies such as a patient with goitre or a patient with rheumatoid arthritis.

Simulated patients

Difficulties in standardising real patients and a lack of availability in some situations led to the development of simulated or standardised patients. These have been used for assessment as well as teaching. The simulated patient, as described in Chapter 25, is usually a lay person who has undergone various levels of training in order to provide a consistent clinical scenario. The examinee interacts with the simulated patient in the same way as if they were taking a history, examining or counselling a real patient. Simulated patients are used most commonly to assess history taking and communication skills or physical examination where no abnormality is found. Simulated patients have also been used to simulate a range of physical findings including, for example, different neurological presentations. The term 'standardised patient' has been used to indicate that the person has been trained to play the role of the patient consistently and according to specific criteria.

Simulators and models

Simulators, from the very basic models used to assess skills such as skin suturing to the more complex interactive whole-body manikins such as SimMan, have been used increasingly in medical training as outlined in Chapter 25. They have an important role to play in assessment. The Harvey cardiac manikin, for example, has been used at an OSCE station to assess skills in cardiac auscultation. Simulators are valuable to assess procedural and practical skills including the insertion of intravenous lines, catheterisation and endoscopy technique. While simulators have played a key role in competence assessment in other fields, notably with airline pilots, simulators have been slow to make an impact in assessment in medicine. The situation has changed rapidly and such devices now play a prominent role in clinical assessment. Indeed in some instances surgeons are allowed to perform a procedure in clinical practice only after they have demonstrated competence on a simulator.

Computer-based simulations

The development of virtual patients is another area where rapid progress has been made. While early computer-based simulations were little more than patient management problems delivered through a computer, computer simulations now include high fidelity models of the patient care environment and the 'patient' responds to the management and therapeutic efforts of the examinee.

THE EXAMINER

In addition to the student and the patient, the third key element in clinical or performance assessment is the examiner. The role of the examiner is to collect evidence about the examinee's behaviour in the context of the assessment and to pass judgement on the examinee's competence or performance. The examiner may be a clinician, another healthcare professional or a simulated patient. After appropriate training simulated patients are, in some situations, particularly in North America, used to assess the student's performance in an OSCE. Other members of the healthcare team frequently contribute to multi-source feedback assessment as described below.

Whatever the assessment method used, it is important to include a number of examiners. A problem with the long case in a traditional clinical examination was over-reliance on the ratings of one or two examiners. In contrast, the OSCE has input from a number of examiners which is a major advantage.

A STUDENT'S PROFILE

A wide range of different learning outcomes or competencies including clinical skills, practical procedures, decision making and problem solving, collaboration and team working and professionalism and attitudes is assessed in a clinical examination. It makes little sense simply to allocate a percentage score for each component and then to sum these to produce a total mark of, for example, 62%. Excellence in carrying out an examination or practical procedure should not compensate for unprofessional behaviour or an inappropriate attitude. The answer is not to agonise over the relative importance of each element of competence and the allocation of a percentage for that element but to produce a competence profile for the examinee. This indicates for each candidate, as shown in Figure 30.2, the domains where their performance is satisfactory or perhaps excellent and those domains or competencies where their performance falls short of what is expected.

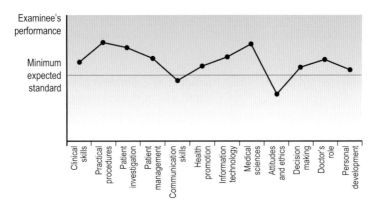

FIG 30.2 An examinee's profile demonstrating competence in some areas but not others.

FEEDBACK

The provision of feedback to the examinee is an important part of a clinical assessment. As discussed in Chapter 2, this should be specific, non-evaluative and timely. It is an essential element of 'assessment for learning' and should guide the learner in their further studies. It is important that when the assessment process is planned, time is allowed for the provision of feedback. The OSCE can be considered as an example of the different approaches that can be adopted:

- Following an OSCE, students' checklists and ratings sheets for each station can be returned to the examinee with the examiner's comments attached.
- Following an OSCE, a meeting with the teacher can be scheduled and the examination is discussed with individuals or the class as a whole.
- During an OSCE, time can be allocated at the end of each station for the provision of feedback from the examiner to the examinee.
- After completion of a station, the examinees review at the following station their own performance at the previous station as recorded on the examiner's checklist and compare this with a model performance as shown on a video recording.

APPROACHES TO CLINICAL AND PERFORMANCE ASSESSMENT

A range of methods have been used to assess the student's or trainee's competence in a controlled clinical environment and to assess how they perform in the work place or real clinical situation.

THE OBJECTIVE STRUCTURED LONG EXAMINATION RECORD (OSLER)

In the traditional long case, the examinee takes a history and examines a patient over a period of up to an hour unobserved by the examiner. Following this the examiner meets with the student and over a 20–30-minute period discusses the patient and the examinee's findings and conclusions. As a replacement for the 'long case' component of a clinical examination, the OSLER was proposed as a more objective and valid assessment of the student's clinical competence (Gleeson 1997).

Over a 30-minute period the examiner uses a structured score sheet to assess the candidate's performance with a patient in the following areas:

- history taking scored in relation to pace and clarity of presentation, communication skills, systematic approach and the establishment of the case facts
- physical examination rated in relation to a systematic approach, examination technique, and the establishment of the correct physical findings
- the ability to determine appropriate investigations for the patient
- the examinee's views on the management of the patient
- the clinical acumen and overall ability to identify and present a satisfactory approach to tackling the patient's problems.

The examiner grades the examinee's performance for each of the areas assessed, taking into account the difficulty of the case, with a rating of 'excellent', 'very good', 'pass', 'bare pass', 'below pass' or 'seriously below pass'. The examiner also records an overall grade for the complete performance.

THE OBJECTIVE STRUCTURED CLINICAL EXAMINATION (OSCE)

The OSCE was introduced in 1975 in response to criticisms about the reliability and validity of the traditional clinical examination. It has been adopted worldwide and is now recognised as the gold standard for the assessment of clinical competence. Students rotate round a series of stations at a predetermined time interval. Each station focuses on one or more aspects of competence, such as history taking, physical examination or carrying out a procedure.

A typical OSCE lasts 2 hours and has 24 stations with 5 minutes being allocated for each station. This allows a wide sample of competencies to be assessed. Some OSCEs have fewer stations with a longer time allocated for each station. In general, however, it is preferable to use shorter stations rather than longer ones as this increases the reliability and validity of the examination. An OSCE with 24 5-minute stations is preferable to an examination with 12 10-minute stations. Where a task cannot be completed in the 5-minute period there are three options:

1. The task can be specified so that it can be completed in 5 minutes.
2. The task can be spread over two linked stations with the first part of the task, for example assessing a patient's record, undertaken at the first station and the subsequent task of counselling the patient assessed at the following station.
3. A station may be duplicated in the circuit to allow students to spend double the set time at the station. This may be useful for a history taking station.

In the OSCE, any subjective bias attributed to an examiner is reduced as the student will encounter a number of examiners during the course of the examination. What is assessed at each station is agreed in advance and a marking schedule is produced which is completed by the examiner. It is important that examiners are fully briefed and trained in advance.

An OSCE should include preferably 'real', simulated or standardised patients, manikins and simulators as each has advantages in what they can offer for the purposes of the assessment. This is not always possible and 'real' patients or simulated patients may dominate in the OSCE.

The content of the examination together with the competencies to be tested is carefully planned on a blueprint in advance of the OSCE. This ensures that the examination tests a range of competencies in relation to different aspects of medical practice. Examples of the types of stations that can be included in an OSCE are given in Appendix 5.

The OSCE offers major attractions as a reliable and valid test of clinical competence. A major advantage is that the format can be easily adapted for use in a wide range of different settings

MINI CLINICAL EVALUATION EXERCISE (MINI-CEX)

In a Mini-CEX the examinee is engaged in an authentic work place based patient encounter. This may be in the in-patient setting, out-patient department or emergency room. The examiner watches the examinee take a focused history, perform relevant parts of the physical examination, provide a diagnosis and present a management plan. The encounter usually lasts about 15–20 minutes and the examiner spends 5 minutes giving the examinee feedback. The performance is scored on a 6- or 9-part scale ranging from below expectations through borderline and meeting expectations to above expectations. The examinee is responsible for the timing of the encounter and for the selection of the patient. The Mini-CEX is repeated on a number of occasions during a clinical attachment with different examiners and different patients.

The Mini-CEX was developed for use in a postgraduate setting but it has been used also in undergraduate education. In this situation the duration of the encounter is often increased from 20 to 40 minutes.

The Mini-CEX has the advantage that it ensures that the clinical skills of the student or trainee are observed in the work place setting by the clinician or trainer and that feedback is given to the learner. The briefing of the examiner and examinee are important.

DIRECT OBSERVATION OF PROCEDURAL SKILLS (DOPS)

This is a variation of the Mini-CEX designed to assess and give feedback on a student's or trainee's procedural skills. As in the Mini-CEX the student or trainee is observed in the work place carrying out the procedure on 'real' patients. The trainee selects the timing and the procedure to be assessed from a prescribed list including, for example, central venous line insertion, arterial blood sampling, electrocardiography and intubation. The examiner may be a clinician or another member of the healthcare team. As with the Mini-CEX, DOPS was designed for use in postgraduate education but has also been applied in undergraduate education.

CASE-BASED DISCUSSION (CbD)

The CbD is used principally in postgraduate training. The trainee selects several case records in which they have made entries regarding patients that they have seen recently. The examiner selects one patient record and explores aspects of it with the trainee. The assessment is designed to assess application of knowledge, decision making and ethical issues as well as medical record keeping. Dimensions assessed include the trainee's clinical assessment of the patient, investigations and referrals, treatment, follow-up and future planning, professionalism and overall clinical judgement. Each dimension is scored on a 6-point scale. Fifteen minutes is allowed for the examination followed by 5 minutes feedback.

MULTI-SOURCE FEEDBACK (MSF) OR 360 DEGREES EVALUATION

MSF has been used for many years in industry and adopted more recently in medicine. It is used in postgraduate and continuing education to assess the practising doctor. Evidence is systematically collected from a number of individuals who are in a legitimate position to make a judgement about the doctor's performance. The individuals may be senior or junior colleagues, other members of the healthcare team, administrators, patients or students. In this way, different perspectives are brought to bear on the evaluation of the doctor. The individual is asked to complete a structured questionnaire relating to the doctor's performance. A '1 to 5' or a '1 to 7' rating scale can be used and comments may also be recorded. The questions asked may be the same or vary for different groups of respondents. Information is collated so that the ratings remain anonymous and the results are fed back to the doctor. The aim is to provide a fair and balanced view of the doctor's behaviour and abilities, particularly in areas such as communication skills, leadership, team working, punctuality and reliability.

MSF is less frequently used in undergraduate education but is sometimes included for assessment purposes in a student's portfolio. This may include peer assessment of professionalism.

MSF offers many advantages, in particular the assessment of the doctor in the real-life practice context. It also has potential disadvantages, in particular the risk of providing damaging and over-harsh feedback.

REFLECT AND REACT

1. The assessment of clinical competence is a central issue in medical education and whatever your role as a teacher, you should be aware of the different approaches and tools available.
2. You may find yourself responsible for the organisation of an OSCE. The OSCE is a flexible tool. See a couple in action then design one to suit your own needs.
3. You may have to serve as an examiner in an OSCE or be the person responsible for providing students with feedback on their performance. Your role may be to advise students or trainees who are about to sit an

OSCE as to how best to prepare for it. Ensure that you are familiar with the examination details.

4. Performance assessment in the work place is particularly challenging. The examiner and examinee both need to be committed to its success. Think about how you might distinguish between competence and performance in your trainees.

EXPLORING FURTHER

IF YOU HAVE A FEW HOURS

Boursicot, K., Etheridge, L., Setna, Z., et al., 2011. Performance in assessment: consensus statement and recommendations from the Ottawa conference. Med. Teach. 33, 370–383.
The conclusions of a group of experts in the area.

Boursicot, K.A.M., Roberts, T.E., Burdick, W.P., 2010. Structured assessments of clinical competence. In: Swanwick, T. (Eds.), Understanding Medical Education: Evidence, Theory and Practice. Wiley-Blackwell, Chichester, pp. 246–258.
Practical advice on planning, running and scoring an OSCE.

Collins, J.P., Harden, R.M., 1998. The use of real patients, simulated patients and simulators in clinical examinations. AMEE Medical Education Guide No. 13. Med. Teach. 20, 508–521.
Patients are a key element in a clinical examination. This is a description of the different ways patients can be represented.

Gleeson, F., 1997. Assessment of clinical competence using the Objective Structured Long Examination Record (OSLER). AMEE Medical Education Guide No. 9. Med. Teach. 19, 7–14.
A description of how the long case can be improved in a clinical examination.

Harden, R.M., Gleeson, F.A., 1979. ASME Medical Education Guide No. 8. Assessment of Medical Competence Using an Objective Structured Clinical Examination (OSCE). ASME, Edinburgh.
An early description of the OSCE but still with much relevance today.

Hill, F., Kendall, K., 2007. Adopting and adapting the mini-CEX as an undergraduate assessment and learning tool. The Clinical Teacher 4, 244–248.
How the Mini-CEX can be used in undergraduate education.

Norcini, J., Burch, V., 2007. Work-place Based Assessment as an Educational Tool. AMEE Medical Education Guide No. 31. AMEE, Dundee.
A description of the range of tools used in work place based assessment.

IF YOU HAVE MORE TIME

Gronlund, N.E., Waugh, C.K., 2009. Assessment of Student Achievement. Pearson, Upper Saddle River, New Jersey.
Chapter 9 in this classic text provides an overview of performance assessment.

Holmboe, E.S., Hawkins, R.E., 2008. Practical Guide to the Evaluation of Clinical Competence. Mosby, St Louis.
A more detailed account of assessment of clinical competence.

Norcini, J., Holmboe, E., 2010. Work-based assessment. In: Cantillon, P., Wood, D. (Eds.), ABC of Learning and Teaching in Medicine. second ed. Wiley-Blackwell, Chichester (Chapter 11).
An introduction to work-based assessment.

Tekian, A., McGuire, C.H., McGaghie, W.C., 1999. Innovative Simulations for Assessing Professional Competence: From Paper-and-Pencil to Virtual Reality. University of Illinois at Chicago Department of Medical Education.
A collection of essays describing innovative applications of simulation technology in assessment and certification in different disciplines.

Portfolio assessment

Portfolio assessment is a response to changes in medical education including the emphasis on professionalism and the need to give students more responsibility for their own learning.

WHAT IS A PORTFOLIO?

A portfolio is a collection of evidence that learning has taken place. It is cumulative in the sense that it contains work collected over a period of time rather than the snapshot view obtained with the traditional examination. It is important to appreciate that a portfolio is different from a logbook. In a portfolio the learner's experiences are recorded but also included are reflections on the experiences and a description of the further learning that has resulted.

The portfolio is likely to contain both quantitative graded evidence as well as qualitative descriptions. Students actively collect and select the material for their portfolio which will provide the examiner with evidence of their learning. Portfolios may include evidence of the practical procedures carried out by the student, videotapes of their clinical experiences, evaluations of their abilities in written assessments and reports by clinicians on the student's clinical attachments. Multi-source feedback from nurses, other members of the healthcare team and patients may be included. The students individualise their portfolio by selecting the evidence relating to their own personal experience. The evidence included in a portfolio is limited only by the degree of the designer's creativity.

WHY PORTFOLIOS?

As described in the previous chapter, in the 1970s there was a switch of emphasis from an assessment of students' knowledge to an assessment of their clinical skills including history taking, physical examination and practical procedures. Tools such as the objective structured clinical examination (OSCE) were developed for this purpose. The more recent move to outcome-based education with an emphasis on learning outcomes such as attitudes, professionalism, reflection and self-assessment created the need for a tool that provided a more valid assessment in these areas. There was a need too for an assessment tool that counteracted a reductionist approach to assessment and which provided a more holistic and overall assessment of a student's competence.

My (RMH) daughter completed two honours degree courses. One was in mathematics and computing and the other in fashion design. She was in no doubt that the assessment method used in her fashion course – portfolio assessment – was much more searching and accurate, and fairer as an assessment of competence in a professional area, than the more traditional examinations used in the mathematics and computing course. Her fashion portfolio contained evidence of work completed during her studies and her reflections on this. It contained evidence of the technical and inter-personal skills she had acquired during her training and demonstrated her understanding of the theory that underpinned the work. Talking with her, the potential value of a portfolio as an assessment tool in medicine was apparent.

Portfolios, which for many years have been used in the arts, are now having a major impact as an assessment tool in medicine. The use of portfolios for learning and assessment has now become widespread in medicine and other healthcare professions. Portfolios are an authentic learning and assessment tool that relates to the work of a doctor and reflects a holistic and integrated approach to medical practice.

ADVANTAGES

Portfolios offer a number of advantages as an assessment tool:

- Outcomes and competencies can be assessed that other tools have difficulty in reaching. These may be skills necessary for life-long learning such as self-assessment, reflection and the adoption of appropriate learning strategies. They provide a tool to assess attitudes and professionalism.
- Portfolios include evidence collected over a period of time and provide an overall and holistic view of a student's competence.
- With the range of quantitative and qualitative evidence included and the triangulation from the different sources of evidence, portfolios provide a comprehensive and reliable interpretation of a student's achievement.
- Portfolios represent a personalised approach to assessment, focusing on what individual students achieve in contrast to the more standardised approach with instruments such as the OSCE.
- As the students go through their course of studies the portfolio integrates learning and assessment and focuses the student's attention on the learning outcomes expected. The student's reflection on the basic sciences relevant to a documented patient encounter reinforces the application of theory to practice.
- The portfolio reinforces a student-centred approach to the curriculum with students being given greater responsibility for their own learning and assessment.

IMPLEMENTING PORTFOLIO ASSESSMENT IN PRACTICE

As an aid to those wishing to design and implement portfolio assessment in their own institution, the late Miriam Friedman Ben David described 10 steps in the portfolio assessment process:

1. *Define the purpose.* It should be made clear whether the portfolio is to be used for summative or formative decisions and how it relates to other elements in the assessment process.

2. *Determine the competencies to be assessed.* Identifying the competencies to be assessed by the portfolio is part of a systematic approach to assessment that ensures that all of the expected learning outcomes are assessed. In particular, the portfolio is valuable in assessing learning outcomes such as attitudes and professionalism and the higher levels of Miller's pyramid.

3. *Define the portfolio content.* Evidence should be included in the portfolio that demonstrates a student's achievement of the learning outcomes to be assessed. Students should be given guidelines as to the type of evidence that is acceptable, but there should be a certain amount of freedom of choice. The type of evidence that is included, the student's comments on it, and their ability to assess their own competence is a measurement of their understanding of the learning outcomes.

   Examples of the type of evidence that might be included are:

   • records of procedures carried out by the student
   • annotated details of patient encounters with details of how they contributed to the student's achievement of the learning outcomes
   • evaluation of the student during clinical clerkships by members of the healthcare team, including nurses and patients
   • videotapes of student interaction with patients.

   A practising doctor's portfolio will comprise a dossier of evidence demonstrating the doctor's continuing education and practice achievements. The evidence included in a portfolio should indicate the student's or practising doctor's progress over time.

4. *Develop a marking system.* Specific criteria may be set out for each of the learning outcomes to be assessed with the portfolio, and a global rating used for the achievement of each outcome:

   4 – excellent, distinguished or superior
   3 – satisfactory, adequate or competent
   2 – minimal borderline or marginal
   1 – unsatisfactory or inadequate.

   Several assessors should review each portfolio with an assessment committee taking a final decision.

5. *Select and train the examiners.* The choice of examiners will depend on the purpose of the assessment and the learning outcomes to be assessed. The examiners should include a range of staff from the basic sciences and clinical medicine. Examiners with less experience can be paired with more senior examiners. The training of the examiners is essential for the success of the programme. Faculty members often appreciate their participation in portfolio examinations as it allows them to get to know more about the individual student and his or her capabilities.

6. *Plan the examination process and timetable.* It is necessary to set a deadline for portfolio submissions. Students' failure to meet the deadline is itself evidence of a lack of professionalism. Time should be scheduled for examiners to read each portfolio and to meet to discuss them.

Portfolio assessment

An opportunity should be provided for them to meet, possibly in pairs, with each student to allow the student to defend the portfolio. Finally, time needs to be set aside for the examiners to discuss each student's performance in order to come to a final decision as to the student's achievement of the learning outcomes assessed.

7. *Student orientation.* Students should be informed in writing about the portfolio assessment process and what is expected of them. In general, the more information given to students the more positive they are about the portfolio.

8. *Develop guidelines for decisions.* If portfolios are used for summative pass/fail decisions, standards need to be specified so that there is no doubt about what constitutes a pass or fail. A decision needs to be made whether poor performance in relation to one outcome assessed can be compensated by good or excellent performance in another area, or whether areas are not compensatory. The medical school in Dundee adopted the approach that a student cannot compensate for deficits in one domain, such as attitudes or professionalism, by a good performance in another domain. Students must achieve the minimum expected standard in every domain.

9. *Establish reliability and validity evidence.* What constitutes good reliable evidence should be agreed prior to the implementation of the portfolio. The degree of reliability may be determined in a pilot study. For example, should there be two pairs of examiners for each portfolio or one pair? Triangulation of the evidence in the portfolio from different sources will increase the validity of the decision reached and guide the faculty as to the use of the portfolio results.

10. *Evaluate the portfolio assessment.* Students' and examiners' opinions on the strengths and weaknesses of portfolios as an assessment tool should be sought. Students' performance with the portfolio assessment should be compared with their performance in an OSCE or written examination and ultimately with their subsequent performance as a doctor. When problems are identified relating to the professionalism or performance of practising doctors, were the same issues identified in their portfolios as students?

REFLECT AND REACT

1. Review the value of portfolios as a tool for student assessment. Which of the advantages listed are applicable to the programme for which you have a responsibility?

2. What could be included in your student's or trainee's portfolio that would provide evidence of their achievement of the expected learning outcomes?

3. If you are an examiner for a portfolio assessment it is important that you fully understand the assessment process and the marking scheme used.

IF YOU HAVE A FEW HOURS

Davis, M.H., Friedman Ben-David, M., Harden, R.M., et al., 2001. Portfolio assessment in medical students' final examinations. Med. Teach. 23, 357–366.
A description of how portfolios can be used as the basis for a final examination in a medical school.

Driessen, E., van Tartwijk, J., van der Vleuten, C., Wass, V., 2007. Portfolios in medical education: why do they meet with mixed success? A systematic review. Med. Educ. 41, 1224–1233.
A description of how portfolios can be used for summative and formative purposes.

Friedman Ben-David, M., Davis, M.H., Harden, R.M., et al., 2001. Portfolios as a Method of Student Aassessment. AMEE Medical Education Guide No. 24. AMEE, Dundee.
Practical advice on the use of portfolios for the purpose of assessment.

van Tartwijk, J., Driessen, E.W., 2010. Portfolios for Assessment and Learning. AMEE Guide No. 45. AMEE, Dundee.
Practical advice on the use of portfolios.

IF YOU HAVE MORE TIME

Buckley, S., Coleman, J., Davidson, I., et al., 2009. The Educational Effects of Portfolios on Undergraduate Student Learning: a Best Evidence Medical Education (BEME) systematic review. AMEE, Dundee.
A summary of the evidence for the educational effects of the use of portfolios in undergraduate education.

Gronlund, N.E., Waugh, C.K., 2009. Assessment of Student Achievement, ninth ed. Pearson, Upper Saddle River, New Jersey.
Chapter 11 describes the value of portfolios as a means of assessment and how they can be scored.

Tochel, C., Haig, A., Hesketh, A., Cadzow, A., et al., 2009. The effectiveness of portfolios for post-graduate assessment and education. BEME Guide No. 12. Med. Teach. 31, 299–318.
A systematic review of the evidence on the effectiveness of portfolios across postgraduate healthcare.

Portfolio assessment

Assessment for admission to medicine and postgraduate training

A range of assessment tools and approaches are available to assist with key selection decisions.

THE IMPORTANCE OF SELECTION

In recent years the methods adopted to select students for admission to medical studies from the large number of applicants have been the focus of attention. There are good reasons for this:

- Owing to low attrition rates, the admission of students to medical studies is almost equivalent to graduating a student. Once students are selected for admission to medicine they will almost certainly complete their medical studies and graduate as a doctor.
- There are political and other pressures to widen access to medical studies and there is wide recognition that doctors should be matched to the community they serve. Some ethnic and social classes may have been disadvantaged in the selection process and this needs to be taken into consideration in the admissions process.
- Once students graduate they are more likely to practise in the geographical area or type of community in which they originally lived.
- The criteria used for selection were based traditionally on academic qualifications. It was assumed that if a student achieved top grades in their studies at school they would automatically develop the competencies expected of a good doctor. This is not necessarily true, and the personal qualities of the potential doctor are recognised to be important as well as their academic qualifications.
- There may be advantages in choosing students whose career goals match the mission of the medical school, for example in relation to a commitment to rural practice.

APPROACHES TO SELECTION FOR ENTRY TO MEDICINE

GRADUATE OR DIRECT FROM SCHOOL ENTRY

In North America, following the Flexner 1910 Report, students were admitted to medical school as graduates following completion of a college course in another subject. In other parts of the world students can enter medical studies direct from school. There has been a move in some medical schools in the UK, Australia and other countries to graduate-only entry. Other schools have maintained a mixed approach accepting both graduates and school leavers. The issue is a controversial one and the arguments for the different approaches are complex. There is no good evidence to indicate that one approach is preferable to the other, but opting to admit students straight from school does have significant financial advantages and there is no evidence that the product is less satisfactory.

A RANGE OF METHODS

Different approaches have been promoted in the selection of students for admission to medicine. Until recently the emphasis has been on academic ability and intellectual achievement. Attention has been paid to selecting an individual who will do well in the medical school examinations rather than to selecting an individual who will become a competent and good doctor. The ability to perform well in tests may simply predict later test scores and not performance as a doctor. The ability to answer MCQs correctly does not necessarily indicate that a student will be a good doctor. This does not mean that a choice has to be made between someone who has a good academic record and someone who will become a good doctor. They are not mutually exclusive.

In general, the criteria for good assessment discussed in Chapter 28 also apply to the selection process. This must be seen to be fair and to be reliable and valid. For this to be so, evidence to support the selection decision should be obtained from a range of sources. The motivation of the student to study medicine must also be taken in to account. Whatever approach to selection is adopted it is important that criteria such as academic ability, personal qualities and ethnicity and any weighting given to the different factors are made explicit. When the entry requirements are considered, attention should be paid to the expected exit learning outcomes of the medical school. Evidence that the student meets minimal requirements relating to each outcome domain prior to entry to medicine is advisable. For example, a required level of competence relating to the communication or attitudinal domains may be specified prior to admission. Learning outcome frameworks that can be used for this purpose are discussed in Chapter 8.

PERFORMANCE AT SCHOOL

Academic achievement and performance at school, as evidenced by A-level achievements in the UK or grade point averages (GPAs) in the USA, have played a major role in decisions about selection. Correlations have been shown between such indicators and students' performance in medical school, particularly in examinations in the early years.

APTITUDE TESTS

Various aptitude tests have been designed to measure a student's ability to develop skills or acquire knowledge. Most have a knowledge component. Examples are the North America College Admission Test (MCAT), the Graduate Australian Medical Admission Test (GAMAT) and the United Kingdom Clinical Aptitude Test (UKCAT).

AUTOBIOGRAPHICAL NARRATIVE

The application form completed by the student may contain useful information about the applicant that will inform the admission decision. The student may be required to provide an autobiographical narrative to justify their motivation to study medicine. Such forms, however, are at risk of fraud and may be written by a third party.

REFERENCES

References may be sought from the student's school, previous employers or individuals with whom the student has been associated. Such letters of recommendation seek to identify personal qualities such as honesty and application. These references are open to bias and tend to be unreliable and ineffective. Laws in relation to disclosure and removal of confidentiality cast additional doubt on their value.

INTERVIEWS

Interviews have been widely used to complement assessment of the student's achievement and aptitude. While questions have been raised about their reliability, they are used to provide evidence that the student has the attributes expected of a future doctor. Structured or semi-structured interviews, where the questions asked are standardised for the candidates and a rating scale is used, have been shown to be more reliable. Interviews, however, are labour intensive and also subject to bias. In one school, when the measurements were taken for refurbishment of the bars in the student union, it was found that the students admitted to the medical school were taller than average. A possible explanation was that the individual in charge of the interview admission process at that time was 6' 6". When interviews are used, training of the interviewer is important.

THE MULTIPLE MINI-INTERVIEW (MMI)

In recent years, there has been increasing emphasis on more objective assessment of students for the purposes of selection with the use of an OSCE approach. The multiple mini-interview (MMI) consists of a series of 5–8-minute testing stations. A rater at each station assesses the student's performance in areas such as ethical decision making, effective communication, empathy, manual dexterity, knowledge of the healthcare system and critical thinking. The MMI requires fewer examiner hours than the traditional type of interview that involved a panel of examiners. The evidence to date is that the MMI has more predictive validity. It provides also a stimulus to prompt admission committees to be more explicit about the qualities they are looking for in applicants.

SELECTION FOR ADMISSION TO SPECIALTY TRAINING

Many of the issues concerning the selection of students to medical studies also apply to the selection of doctors for postgraduate training. Undergraduate performance and interviews play a significant part in the process. Dean's letters and other references are often used but again their reliability is suspect.

Not much attention has been paid to matching doctors on graduation with the career for which they are best suited. The skills expected of a surgeon will differ in some respects from the abilities and characteristics expected of a doctor working in public health.

REFLECT AND REACT

1. You should familiarise yourself with the selection procedure in your institution. To what extent does this reflect the attributes expected of a future doctor?
2. To what extent do the principles of good assessment described in Chapter 28 apply to the selection process in your institution?
3. If you are involved in a selection committee, an interview panel or as an assessor in an MMI you should ensure that you are familiar with the rules and complete the necessary training.
4. Consider how social accountability of universities and training organisations should be reflected in the selection process and the widening of access.

EXPLORING FURTHER

IF YOU HAVE A FEW HOURS

Eva, K.W., Rosenfield, J., Reiter, H.I., et al., 2004. An admissions OSCE: the multiple mini-interview. Med. Educ. 38, 314–326.
A description of this relatively new approach.

Harris, S., Owen, C., 2007. Discerning quality: using the multiple mini-interview in student selection for the Australian National University Medical School. Med. Educ. 41, 234–241.
A description of the use of the MMI in the selection of students in one school.

McGaghie, W.C., 2002. Student selection. In: Norman, G.R., van der Vleuten, C.P.M., Newble, D.I. (Eds.), International Handbook of Research in Medical Education. Kluwer Academic Publishers, London (Chapter 10).
A useful summary of medical student selection criteria and some of the methods adopted.

Prideaux, D., Roberts, C., Eva, K., et al., 2011. Assessment for selection for the health care professions and specialty training: consensus statement and recommendations from the Ottawa 2010 conference. Med. Teach. 33, 215–223.
Recommendations from an expert group on assessment for selection in medicine.

Evaluating the curriculum

33

Curriculum evaluation is an essential part of the educational process. The focus in curriculum evaluation is on quality improvement.

THE IMPORTANCE OF EVALUATION

The earlier chapters in this section are concerned with the evaluation of the student. In this chapter we look at the evaluation of the medical school or educational organisation and the curriculum in the institution. This is important for a number of reasons:

- With the current emphasis on quality assurance it is important to ascertain whether the curriculum and the teaching are fit for purpose.
- Curriculum development is an ongoing iterative process, which requires to be informed by an evaluation of current practice and with feedback as to problems identified.
- There is a move to recognise excellence in education in medical schools as well as excellence in research.

LEVELS OF EVALUATION

An evaluation of the education programme can be conceptualised at different levels:

- At the macro level the mission of the medical school and the extent to which the school is achieving its overall aims should be examined.
- At the micro level the elements of the curriculum should be evaluated. These include the learning outcomes, the teaching, learning and assessment methods, the educational strategies, the education environment, the management of the curriculum and the engagement with students and staff.

ASSESSMENT OF THE MEDICAL SCHOOL/INSTITUTION

The educational programme within the institution and the management structure should be evaluated as described below. It is important also to take a broader look at the institution and its achievements. Are the aims as set out in the mission of the institution appropriate and are they being achieved?

213

THE MISSION OF THE SCHOOL

An aspect of the mission of a medical school that has attracted attention is the social responsibility and accountability of the school. A school should not be an ivory tower but should be regarded as excellent only if significant attention is paid to its social accountability and how it relates to the community that it serves. Boelen and Woollard (2009) have argued that for a school to be socially responsible it needs to have a commitment to respond to the priority health needs of citizens and society. The impact of the educational institution on society and the public good should be part of the assessment of its success. It has been shown that the most research-active medical schools demonstrate the least social responsibility. Some schools see as their mission the development of future leaders or researchers.

THE SCHOOL'S GRADUATES

Another factor in the assessment of a medical school is the consideration and attention paid to the continuum of medical education and the further professional development of its graduates. Has the school collaborated in the development of its curriculum with the range of stakeholders, including patients and those in the health service responsible for employing the doctors?

INTERNATIONAL DIMENSION

With increased globalisation in medicine and medical care, the extent to which the medical school is adequately equipping its graduates as citizens of the world should be evaluated. Graduates should have a sound knowledge of global issues, the skills for working in an international context and the values of a global citizen.

CURRICULUM EVALUATION

DEFINITION

Curriculum evaluation can be defined as 'a deliberate act of enquiry which sets out with the intention of allowing people concerned with an educational event to make rigorous, informed judgements and decisions about it so that appropriate development may be facilitated' (Coles and Grant 1985).

AIMS OF CURRICULUM EVALUATION

The evaluation of a curriculum can have different purposes:

- Demonstration of the achievement of the minimum standards expected by an accrediting body such as the General Medical Council in the UK, the Liaison Committee on Medical Education (LCME) in the USA or the Australian Medical Council (AMC) in Australia. The World Federation for Medical Education (WFME) has set out minimum standards for educational programmes at undergraduate, postgraduate and continuing education levels.

- Establishing that the programme as set out ('the planned curriculum') is in fact happening ('the received curriculum'). There is often a gap between what is set out on paper and what happens in practice.
- As an essential requirement for curriculum development. Without an evaluation of the curriculum there can be no informed curriculum development. Curriculum evaluation should be concerned not simply with a measurement of the success or failure of a curricular initiative but be a more complex assessment that provides a fuller understanding of the education process. Parlett and Hamilton (1975) described this as 'illuminative evaluation'.
- The assessment of a curriculum change. A better understanding of a change made to the curriculum can be sought and the extent to which it has been effective measured. The difference between curriculum evaluation and research is sometimes questioned. As argued by Kelly (2004), curriculum evaluation becomes part of curriculum research. In the context of research, the findings of the evaluation must be examined from a generalisable perspective. Curriculum planning and evaluation can be seen as hypotheses to be tested.
- A comparison between and understanding of education programmes in institutions in different countries or with different approaches and admission policies. Such information is useful in the context of student mobility as well as for use in research in medical education.
- The provision of information for potential students. A curriculum evaluation can provide information not only on the excellence of the education programme in a medical school but also on its character, and this might inform a student's choice of medical school. The publication by the Higher Education Funding Councils in the UK of the ratings of the education programmes in medical schools was associated with significant changes in the pattern of schools to which students applied to be admitted.

APPROACHES TO CURRICULUM EVALUATION

A number of frameworks can be used in curriculum evaluation. Here we describe the 'ten questions' framework and the Kirkpatrick four levels of evaluation.

THE TEN QUESTIONS

The ten questions to be addressed in the planning of a curriculum, as described in Chapter 11, can be used also as a framework for a curriculum evaluation. Examples are given of the issues to be addressed relating to each question.

1. *The needs which the medical school aims to meet.* The evaluation of the mission of the medical school is discussed earlier in the chapter.

2. *Learning outcomes.*
    - How is the move to outcome-based education (OBE) interpreted and implemented in the medical school? Teachers have very different perceptions of the significance of learning outcomes and this may influence the delivery of the education programme.
    - A framework to assess the implementation of OBE in a medical school is described in Chapter 9.

3. *The curriculum content.*
   - What content is addressed in the curriculum and how does this relate to the stated learning outcomes? How are new subjects such as genetics addressed alongside more traditional subjects?
   - What constitutes the core curriculum?
   - Is there a danger of information overload and how is this addressed?

4. *Sequence and organisation.*
   - What consideration has been given to the organisation and sequencing of content within the curriculum?
   - To what extent is there exposure to clinical experiences early in the programme and to the basic medical sciences later?

5. *Educational strategies.*
   The 'SPICES' model as described in Chapter 11 is a useful tool to analyse the curriculum and the educational strategies adopted:
   - Student-centred/Teacher-centred
   - Problem-based/Information-based
   - Integrated/Discipline-based
   - Community orientated/Hospital orientated
   - Electives/Core plus uniform
   - Systematic/Opportunistic

   Each dimension represents a continuum on which the school will be placed somewhere between the two extremes.

6. *Teaching and learning methods and opportunities.*
   - Is there a grid or blueprint that relates the expected learning outcomes to the courses in the curriculum and the available learning opportunities?
   - To what extent has there been a move to more 'authentic learning'?
   - What is the balance between technology-based and more traditional approaches to learning?
   - To what extent is collaborative or peer-to-peer learning encouraged and developed?
   - To what extent are the international dimensions to learning incorporated?

7. *Assessment.*
   - To what extent is assessment blueprinted against the learning outcomes?
   - To what extent is the rich range of tools now available harnessed to assess students' competence?
   - Is there a measure of the students' progression through the curriculum?
   - Is there adequate feedback to the students and teachers?

8. *Educational environment.*
   - How can the education environment in the medical school be characterised and is this in line with the expected learning outcomes?
   - Has the education environment been measured using a tool as described in Chapter 18?

9. *Communication about the curriculum.*
   - How is the information about the medical curriculum communicated to staff, students and other stakeholders?
   - Is a curriculum map available?

10. *Management.*
   - Does the management structure support the implementation of the curriculum?
   - Are the roles of the teachers defined and matched to their abilities?
   - How is teaching recognised and rewarded within the medical school?
   - Is a staff development programme implemented and how are teachers kept up-to-date with advances in medical education and in their own specialty?
   - What sort of quality assurance processes are in place?

KIRKPATRICK'S FOUR LEVELS OF EVALUATION

Kirkpatrick described four levels for assessing the effectiveness of training. Although the model was developed for use in a business context it has been widely applied in medical education.

Each successive level in the model provides a more precise measure of the effectiveness of the educational programme but requires a more rigorous and time-consuming analysis. Kirkpatrick suggests that evaluation can begin at the first level and, as time and resources allow, move to the higher levels (Fig. 33.1).

Level 1: Opinion/reaction. Evaluation at this level examines how participants in the education programme react to it. Are they satisfied? Do they like or dislike it? Does it meet their needs?

Level 2: Competence/learning. This level moves beyond the learner's satisfaction, and the extent to which there is a difference in the learner's knowledge, skills or attitudes is assessed. Students' performance in written or clinical assessments is studied and taken as evidence of the effectiveness of the education programme.

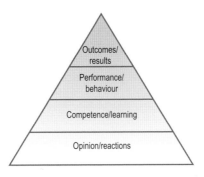

FIG 33.1 Kirkpatrick's four levels.

Level 3: Performance/behaviour transfer. Changes in the learner's behaviour are studied at this level. As a result of the education programme do students communicate more effectively in their day-to-day contacts with patients? Do students apply their knowledge of the basic sciences to understand better the pathophysiology of patients they encounter?

Level 4: Outcome/results. This level, in the context of Kirkpatrick's work, measures the success of a training programme in terms of the business results. Did sales increase after training was completed? In medical education the question is whether the training of the doctor affects medical practice. Does the training in cardiac auscultation and the interpretation of murmurs, for example, reduce the need for laboratory investigations of patients? Does education of doctors about hypertension reduce the incidence of side effects in patients presenting with raised blood pressure?

UNDERTAKING A CURRICULUM EVALUATION

Undertaking a curriculum evaluation involves:

- Clarifying the purpose of the evaluation. A number of different aims are mentioned earlier in the chapter.
- Deciding the approach to be adopted. The 'ten questions' model and the Kirkpatrick four levels approach are described.
- Engaging the stakeholders. These include the curriculum committee, the teachers, the students, other health professionals, future employers and the public.
- Planning the methods to be used. These almost certainly will include qualitative and quantitative methods.
- Allocating responsibilities for the implementation of the evaluation and the necessary resources to carry it out.
- Planning how the results will be communicated and how action will be taken as a result of the evaluation.

REFLECT AND REACT

1. Are you aware of the stated mission for your medical school or educational body? How successfully is this achieved?
2. What purposes described for curriculum evaluation are relevant to your situation?
3. What steps are taken to evaluate your curriculum and are all the stakeholders involved? Is effective use made of the results of the evaluation?

IF YOU HAVE A FEW HOURS

Boelen, C., Woollard, B., 2009. Social accountability and accreditation: a new frontier for educational institutions. Med. Educ. 43, 887–894.

Coles, C.R., Grant, J.G., 1985. Curriculum evaluation in medical and healthcare education. Med. Educ. 19, 405–422.
A description of what is meant by curriculum evaluation in medical education.

Harden, R.M., 1986. Ten questions to ask when planning a course or curriculum. Med. Educ. 20, 356–365.
A description of the ten questions to be asked when planning a curriculum.

IF YOU HAVE MORE TIME

Berk, R.A., 2006. Thirteen Strategies to Measure College Teaching. A Consumer's Guide to Rating Scale Construction, Assessment, and Decision Making for Faculty, Administrators, and Clinicians. Stylus Publishing, Sterling, Virginia.
An amusingly written account of how to assess the effectiveness of teaching.

Kelly, A.V., 2004. The Curriculum: Theory and Practice, fifth ed. SAGE Publications, London.
A useful account of the purpose, approaches and theory underpinning curriculum evaluation.

Kirkpatrick, D., Kirkpatrick, J., 2006. Evaluating Training Programs: The Four Levels, third ed. Berrett-Koehler, San Francisco.
A description of the Kirkpatrick four levels of evaluation.

Parlett, M., Hamilton, D., 1975. Evaluation as illumination. In: Tawney, D. (Ed.), Curriculum Evaluation Today: Trends and Implications. Schools Council Research Studies, Macmillan, London.
A classic description of illuminative education.

SECTION 6
TODAY'S TEACHER AND TOMORROW'S DOCTORS

'Everyone who remembers his own educational experience remembers teachers, not methods and techniques. The teacher is the kingpin of the educational situation.'
Sidney Hook

OVERVIEW

Chapter **34** The changing role of the teacher
- The teacher is a key factor in the education of tomorrow's doctors
- The good teacher embodies a range of abilities
- The teacher should adapt to changes in medical education
- The abilities required of a teacher can be learned
- This book can help the teacher to develop the necessary skills

The changing role of the teacher 34

THE TEACHER IS A KEY FACTOR IN THE EDUCATION OF TOMORROW'S DOCTORS

This book is about the teacher and the essential role the teacher plays in the education of tomorrow's doctors. The achievement of the learning outcomes by the student and the sort of doctor they become can to a large measure be attributed to the teachers who have served as their role models and who have been responsible for their undergraduate and postgraduate training. The teachers, as we have discussed in the Preface and in Chapter 1, are a medical school's most important asset.

THE GOOD TEACHER EMBODIES A RANGE OF ABILITIES

Teaching is a complex activity that requires a range of abilities of the teacher as described in Chapter 2. This includes not only the teacher's mastery of the content area but also the technical competencies necessary to serve as an information provider, a role model, a facilitator of learning, a curriculum planner, an assessor and a resource developer. As a professional, the teacher requires a basic understanding of the underpinning educational principles and an appropriate attitude and passion for teaching. The teacher should be an enquirer into his or her own competence and keep themselves up-to-date with developments in the field. This is summarised in the equation:

$$\text{An excellent teacher (ET)} = (\text{Ieq} + \text{Req} + \text{Feq} + \text{Aeq} + \text{Ceq} + \text{Leq}) \times (\text{S} \times \text{E} \times \text{D} \times \text{T}) \times (\text{P})$$

where I is information provider, R is role model, F is facilitator, A is assessor, C is curriculum planner, L is learning resource developer, e is extent, q is quality, S is scientific principles, E is ethics and attitudes, D is decision making, T is team working and P is personal development.

With the necessary skills, teaching is not a chore; it can be an enjoyable experience and can be rewarding and fun. The good teacher will have a passion for teaching that will help to motivate and inspire students and trainees.

THE TEACHER SHOULD ADAPT TO CHANGES IN MEDICAL EDUCATION

Important changes are taking place not only in medical practice but also in how the doctor of tomorrow is trained. The changes are outlined in Table 34.1. They reflect changes in the students admitted to medical studies, changes in educational thinking and learning technologies and changes in public expectations. These changes impose new demands on the teacher with a change in emphasis from the teacher as an information provider to the teacher as the facilitator of learning. The teacher must respond to changes in what is expected in terms of the learning outcomes. The teacher has also to be familiar with the application of the new technologies to education.

Table 34.1 *Changes in medical education*	
Past	**Present and Future**
Emphasis on the process and the methods of teaching and learning	Emphasis on the product and the learning outcomes
Learning dominated by mastery of basic and clinical science theory	Authentic learning with theory related to real-life situations and problems
Clinical experiences introduced later in the course	Clinical experiences introduced early in the course
Learning through lectures and hospital-based clinical teaching	A mixed economy including e-learning and simulation and learning in ambulatory and community-based settings
Teachers take responsibility for the education	Students actively engage in their own learning
Uniform or standard education programme	Teaching personalised to the needs of individual students
Curriculum content compartmentalised and discipline based	Curriculum content integrated
Education based within the medical profession	Inter-professional education and learning to work in teams
A competitive environment with students learning as individuals	Students collaborate and learn together
Assessment prioritises mastery of fact	Assessment rewards skills and attitudes
Emphasis is on being correct, with mistakes and errors ignored	Learning from mistakes and errors in practice
Education decisions made on the teacher's prejudice and personal experience	Education decisions informed by the best evidence available

THE ABILITIES REQUIRED OF A TEACHER CAN BE LEARNED

Expertise in medicine or in a content area is not necessarily associated with the skills required to teach the subject to students or trainees. While a good teacher may naturally have the necessary skills and passion to teach others, some of the required skills have to be learned. Everyone can learn to be a teacher. With appropriate training, the good teacher can become an excellent teacher and the poor teacher can become a good teacher.

THIS BOOK CAN HELP THE TEACHER TO DEVELOP THE NECESSARY SKILLS

Teachers who fail to keep up-to-date with education developments will no longer have a meaningful role to play in the education of students (Fig. 34.1).

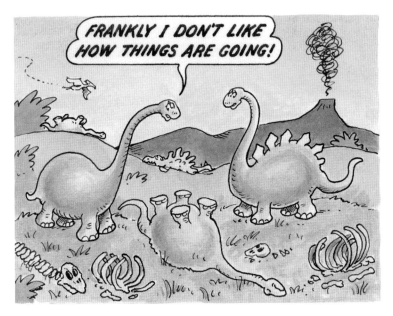

FIG 34.1   Medical teachers need to be able to adapt to change.

This book helps the teacher to keep up-to-date by providing practical guidance on the competencies necessary to deliver a high quality education programme. It introduces the teacher to their responsibilities in curriculum planning, in implementing a teaching and learning programme and in the assessment of students and provides the necessary theoretical underpinning.

FURTHER READING

MEDICAL EDUCATION

Calman, K.C., 2006. Medical Education: Past, Present and Future. Elsevier, Edinburgh.

Carter, Y., Jackson, N. (Eds.), 2009. Medical Education and Training: From Theory to Delivery. Oxford University Press, Oxford.

Cooke, M., Irby, D.M., O'Brien, B.C., 2010. Educating Physicians: A Call for Reform of Medical School and Residency. Jossey-Bass, San Francisco.

Dent, J.A., Harden, R.M. (Eds.), 2009. A Practical Guide for Medical Teachers, third ed. Elsevier, Edinburgh.

Dornan, T., Mann, K., Scherpbier, A., Spencer, J. (Eds.), 2011. Medical Education Theory and Practice. Elsevier, Edinburgh.

McKimm, J., Swanwick, T., 2010. Clinical Teaching Made Easy. Quay Books Ltd, London.

Norman, G.R., Van der Vleuten, C.P.M., Newble, D.I. (Eds.), 2002. International Handbook of Research in Medical Education Part One and Two. Kluwer Academic Publishers, Dordrecht.

Shields, H.M., 2011. A Medical Teacher's Manual for Success: Five Simple Steps. The John Hopkins University Press, Baltimore.

Swanwick, T. (Ed.), 2010. Understanding Medical Education: Evidence, Theory and Practice. ASME/Wiley-Blackwell, Chichester.

GENERAL

Bransford, J.D., Brown, A.L., Cocking, R.R. (Eds.), 2000. How People Learn: Brain, Mind, Experience and School. National Academy Press, Washington DC.

Fink, L.D., 2003. Creating Significant Learning Experiences. Jossey-Bass, San Francisco.

Marzano, R. (Ed.), 2010. On Excellence in Teaching. Solution Tree Press, Bloomington, Indiana.

Pratt D D and Associates, 2005. Five Perspectives on Teaching in Adult and Higher Education. Krieger Publishing Company, Malabar, Florida.

Sotto, E., 2007. When Teaching becomes Learning, second ed. Continuum International Publishing Group, London.

APPENDICES

APPENDIX I

AMEE MEDICAL TEACHER'S CHARTER (modified from the Charter for Teachers produced by the Australian Curriculum Studies Association)

1. Medical teachers believe in the power of medical education across the continuum from undergraduate through postgraduate to continuing education to make a difference to the practice of medicine and to the healthcare of communities throughout the world.
2. As teachers we are committed to give our students and trainees the best education possible for them to lead fulfilling, purposeful and productive lives as healthcare professionals.
3. Medical teachers set high standards for every learner and respond to individual needs. We challenge students to be all that they can be as doctors, to set demanding goals for themselves and to work as effective members of the healthcare team.
4. We have expertise in teaching and learning and provide opportunities that engage each student's capacity to learn. We help our students to achieve the learning outcomes expected of them.
5. We provide a stimulating and supportive learning environment. We help to create medical school and postgraduate education settings that welcome students and trainees and foster the achievement of the prescribed learning outcomes including appropriate attitudes and professionalism.
6. We inspire learners to discover the joy of learning, drawing them into a world of knowledge, skills, ideas and creativity. Our ambition for all is a life-long engagement with learning.
7. Our practice as a teacher reflects the essential balance between conserving and renewing the best of current teaching practice and anticipating and developing new approaches. In achieving this we work in partnership with colleagues and other professions.
8. We act and make decisions in relation to our teaching based on our judgement and on the evidence relating to good practice in the area.
9. We take responsibility for advancing the professionalism and scholarship of medical education.
10. The medical teaching profession sets itself demanding standards. We act with judgement, integrity and respect to build the trust and confidence of all the stakeholders including the public, the government, the healthcare professions and the learners.

APPENDIX 2

COMPONENTS OF A STUDY GUIDE (reproduced with permission from Harden, Laidlaw & Hesketh, 1999, AMEE Guide No.16 Study Guides: Their use and preparation.)

	Essential	Possible	Omit
A Management of learning			
1. Overview of topic or course	☐	☐	☐
2. Learning outcomes	☐	☐	☐
3. Prerequisites	☐	☐	☐
4. Timetable	☐	☐	☐
5. Learning strategies	☐	☐	☐
6. Learning opportunities	☐	☐	☐
7. Assessment	☐	☐	☐
8. Staff contacts	☐	☐	☐
9. Personal comments by authors	☐	☐	☐
B Activities			
1. Interaction with lectures and resource material	☐	☐	☐
2. Application of theory to clinical practice	☐	☐	☐
3. Self-assessment exercises	☐	☐	☐
4. Record of achievement or portfolio	☐	☐	☐
5. Personal information bank	☐	☐	☐
6. Student comments on the guide	☐	☐	☐
C Information			
a) Previously published			
1. Reference to texts and journals	☐	☐	☐
2. Quotations from texts and journal	☐	☐	☐
3. Longer extracts from texts and journals	☐	☐	☐
4. Complete texts or articles	☐	☐	☐
b) New information			
1. Short comments on the topic	☐	☐	☐
2. Short notes	☐	☐	☐
3. Key or core information	☐	☐	☐
4. More extended account of the topic	☐	☐	☐
5. Glossary, definitions or list of terms used	☐	☐	☐

APPENDIX 3

THE CLINICAL PRESENTATIONS THAT PROVIDE A FRAMEWORK FOR THE CURRICULUM IN TASK-BASED LEARNING
(reproduced with permission from Harden et al, 2000, Medical Education 34: 391–397.)

1. **Pain**
   Pain in the leg on walking
   Acute abdominal pain
   Loin pain and dysuria
   Joint pain
   Back and neck pain
   Indigestion
   Headache
   Cancer pain
   Earache
2. **Bleeding and bruising**
   Bruising easily
   Pallor
   Haemoptysis
   Vomiting blood
   Rectal bleeding
   Blood in urine
   Anaemia
   Post-operative bleeding
3. **Fever and infection**
   Chest infection
   Rash and fever
   Urethral discharge
   Pyrexia of unknown origin
   Immunisation
   Sweating
   Hypothermia
   Sepsis
4. **Altered consciousness**
   Immobility
   Falls
   Collapse
   Confusion
   Dizziness
   Fits
5. **Paralysis and impaired mobility**
   Loss of power on one side
   Tremor
   Peripheral neuropathy
   Muscle weakness
   Immobility
   Falling over
6. **Lumps, bumps and swelling**
   Lump in the neck
   Lump in groin
   Lump in breast
   Swollen scrotum
   Joint swelling
   Swollen ankles
   Skin lump
7. **Nutrition/weight**
   Thirsty and losing weight
   Difficulty swallowing
   Weight loss
   Seriously overweight
8. **Change in body function**
   Wheezing
   Pleural effusion
   Shortness of breath
   Cough
   Change in bowel habit
   Cannot pass urine
   Incontinence
   Raised blood pressure
   Palpitations
9. **Skin problems**
   Skin rash
   Itching
   Psoriasis
   Mole growing bigger/bleeding

Blistering
Photosensitivity
Bedsore
Jaundice
Burn
Wound

10. **Life threatening/Accident and Emergency**
Shock
Involvement in accident
Fracture

11. **Eyes**
Loss of vision
Painful red eyes
Squinting in child
Foreign body in child

12. **Ear, nose and throat**
Ringing in ear
Going deaf
Earache
Sore throat
Hoarseness
Stuffy nose

13. **Behaviour**
Anger
Anxiety
Phobias
Drug addiction
Suicide
Sleep problems
Bereavement

Alcohol dependence
Schizophrenia
Tiredness
Depression
Adolescence

14. **Reproductive problems**
Pre-menstrual syndrome
Infertility
Normal pregnancy
Menstrual problems
Contraception
Sterilisation
Smear results
Painful intercourse

15. **The child**
Child abuse
Down's syndrome
Prematurity
Poor feeding
Failure to thrive
Respiratory distress syndrome
Developmental delay
Sudden infant death syndrome/
near miss

16. **Priority setting, decision making and audit**
Dying patient
Population screening
Waiting lists
Triage
Acute vs chronic

APPENDIX 4

A PAGE FROM A STUDY GUIDE, 'LEARNING PAEDIATRICS: A TRAINING GUIDE FOR SENIOR HOUSE OFFICERS' (reproduced with permission from Harden, Laidlaw & Hesketh 1999 AMEE Guide No.16 Study Guides: Their use and preparation.)

Therapy

Strict schedules governing oral intake are not helpful. Discuss with nursing and medical staff when oral fluids or diet should be increased or reintroduced.

Black's *Paediatric Emergencies* has several useful sections.
• Appendix 3, p766-769 (water and electrolyte requirements)
• Appendix 5, p773-755 (advice on necessary maintenance fluids)

For an overview of home-based oral rehydration for diarrhoea, Almroth & Lathham, *Lancet*, Mar 1995; 345(8951) 709-711.

A Meyes, Modern management of acute diarrhoea and dehydration in children. *Am Fam Phys*, Apr 1995: 57(5): 1103-1118, may also give you some ideas.

Teamwork

Speak to colleagues in the local Public Health Department. Discuss infection-control policies and notification of diseases.

Experienced nursing staff may help you decide on the best method of rehydration. Remember – you can always reassess cases after a few hours and review your decisions.

Professional development

Do you know how to prevent cross contamination?

With each case, consider what measures may be required e.g. hand washing alone, or additional gloves, masks and gowns.

Think why a child is being barrier nursed. Is it to protect the patient or the staff/other patients/environment?

Look at the local infection-control policy for guidance.

Microbiology in Clinical Practice (p602-607) contains a short section on different standards of isolation, with suggested isolation procedures.

APPENDIX 5

EXAMPLES OF OSCE STATIONS

- History taking from a patient who presents with a problem, e.g. abdominal pain.
- History taking to elucidate a diagnosis, e.g. hypothyroidism.
- Educating a patient about management, e.g. use of inhaler for asthma.
- Advice to a patient and his wife, e.g. on discharge from hospital with a myocardial infarction.
- Explanation to a patient about tests and procedures, e.g. endoscopy.
- Communication with other members of healthcare teams, e.g. brief to nurse with regard to a terminally ill patient.
- Communication with relatives, e.g. informing a wife that her husband has bronchial carcinoma.
- Physical examination of system or part of body, e.g. examination of hands.
- Physical examination to follow up a problem identified, e.g. congestive cardiac failure.
- Physical examination to help confirm or refute a diagnosis, e.g. thyrotoxicosis.
- A diagnostic procedure, e.g. ophthalmoscopy.
- Written communication, e.g. writing referral letter or discharge letter.
- Interpretation of findings and follow-up action, e.g. charts, laboratory reports or findings documented in patient's records.
- Management, e.g. writing a prescription or commentary on a prescription.
- Critical appraisal, e.g. review of published article or pharmaceutical advertisement.
- Management of errors, e.g. meet with a senior hospital administrator to follow up a letter of complaint from a patient who complains that her weight as recorded was not her correct weight and initiate the action to be taken.

APPENDIX 6

THE LEARNING OUTCOMES FOR A COMPETENT PRACTITIONER BASED ON THE THREE-CIRCLE MODEL (reproduced with permission from Harden et al, 1999, AMEE Guide No 14: Outcome based education Part 5.)

A **What the doctor is able to do – 'doing the right thing'**

Technical Intelligences

Clinical skills	Practical procedures	Patient investigation	Patient management	Health promotion and disease prevention	Communication	Appropriate information handling skills
History Physical examination Interpretation of findings Formulation of action plan	Cardiology Dermatology Endocrinology Gastroenterology Haematology Musculo skeletal Nervous system Ophthalmology Otolaryngology	General principles Clinical Imaging Biochemical medicine Haematology Immunology	General principles Drugs Surgery Psychological Physiotherapy Radiotherapy Social Nutrition Emergency medicine Acute care	Recognition of causes of threats to health and individuals at risk Implementation where appropriate of basics of prevention Collaboration with other health professionals in health promotion and disease prevention	With patient With relatives With colleagues With agencies With media/press Teaching Managing Patient advocate Mediation and negotiation By telephone In writing	Patient records Accessing data sources Use of computers Implementation of professional guidelines Personal records (log books, portfolios)

	B How the doctor approaches their practice – 'doing the thing right'		C The doctor as a professional – 'the right person doing it'	
Intellectual Intelligences	*Emotional Intelligences*	*Analytical and creative Intelligences*	*Personal Intelligences*	
Understanding of social, basic and clinical sciences and underlying principles	Appropriate attitudes, ethical understanding and legal responsibilities	Appropriate decision making skills, and clinical reasoning and judgement	Role of the doctor within the health service	Personal development
Normal structure and function Normal behaviour The life cycle Pathophysiology Psychosocial model of illness Pharmacology and Clinical Pharmacology Public health medicine Epidemiology Preventative medicine and health prevention Education Health economics	Attitudes Understanding of ethical principles Ethical standards Legal responsibilities Human rights issues Respect for colleagues Medicine in multicultural societies Awareness of psycho-social issues Awareness of economic issues Acceptance of responsibility to contribute to advance of medicine Appropriate attitude to professional institution and health service bodies	Clinical reasoning Evidence-based medicine Critical thinking Research method Statistical understanding Creativity/ resourcefulness Coping with uncertainty Prioritisation	Understanding of healthcare systems Understanding of clinical responsibilities and role of doctor Acceptance of code of conduct and required personal attributes Appreciation of doctor as researcher Appreciation of doctor as mentor or teacher Appreciation of doctor as manager including quality control Appreciation of doctor as member of multi-professional team and of roles of other healthcare professionals	Self learner Self awareness Enquires into own competence Emotional awareness Self confidence Self regulation Self care Self control Adaptability to change Personal time management Motivation Achievement drive Commitment Initiative Career choice

APPENDIX 7

QUESTIONNAIRE USED TO ASSESS THE TEACHER'S PERCEPTION OF THE IMPORTANCE OF THE 12 ROLES AND THEIR CURRENT PERSONAL COMMITMENT AND PREFERRED PERSONAL FUTURE COMMITMENT TO EACH ROLE (reproduced with permission from Harden & Crosby 2000, AMEE Guide No. 20 The good teacher is more than a lecturer: the 12 roles of the teacher.)

Teacher's role	Importance to medical school teaching programme					Current personal commitment					Preferred personal future commitment				
	None 1	Little 2	Some 3	Considerable 4	Great 5	None 1	Little 2	Some 3	Considerable 4	Great 5	None 1	Little 2	Some 3	Considerable 4	Great 5
Information provider															
1 Lecturer in classroom setting															
2 Teacher in clinical or practical class setting															
Role model															
3 On-the-job model (e.g. in clinics, ward rounds etc)															
4 Role model in the teaching setting															
Facilitator															
5 Mentor, personal adviser or tutor to a student or group of students															
6 Learning facilitator, e.g. supporting students' learning in problem-based learning small groups, in the laboratory, in the integrated practical class sessions or in the clinical setting															
Examiner															
7 Planning or participating in formal examinations of students															
8 Curriculum evaluator - evaluation of the teaching programme and the teachers															
Planner															
9 Curriculum planner, participating in overall planning of the curriculum through curriculum planning committees															
10 Course organiser, responsibility for planning and this may, for example, relate to one system or one theme, or to a special study module															
Resource developer															
11 Production of study guides to support the students' learning in the course															
12 Developing learning resource materials in the form of computer programmes, videotape or print which can be used as adjuncts to the lectures and other sessions															

APPENDIX 8

THE COMPETENCIES AND THE ROLES OF THE TEACHER

Teacher role	Technical competencies			Scientific principles			Ethics and attitudes			Decision making			Professionalism		
	?	+	+++	?	+	+++	?	+	+++	?	+	+++	?	+	+++
Information provider															
Role model															
Facilitator															
Assessor															
Curriculum planner															
Resource developer															

APPENDIX 9

SUMMARY OF VARIOUS POINTS IN THE CONTINUUM BETWEEN A PROBLEM-BASED APPROACH AND AN INFORMATION-ORIENTATED APPROACH.

'Rul' is the rules or Principles to be Learned. 'Eg' is the Problem or Clinical example addressed by the Student. (Reproduced with permission. First published in Harden & Davis, Medical Teacher, 1998, 20: 317–322.)

		Terminology	Description	Example
1	Rul (Th)	Theoretical learning.	Information provided about the theory.	Traditional lecture. Standard textbook.
2	Rul PT	Problem-orientated learning.	Practical information provided.	Lecture with practical information. Protocols or guidelines.
3	Rul → Eg	Problem-assisted learning.	Information provided with the opportunity to apply it to practical examples.	Lecture followed by practical or clinical experience. Book with problems or experiences included.
4	Eg	Problem-solving learning.	Problem-solving related to specific examples.	Case discussions and some activities in practical classes.
5	Rul → Eg → Rul	Problem-focused learning.	Information is provided followed by a problem. The principles of the subject are then learned.	Introductory or foundation courses or lecture. Information in study guide.
6	Rul → Eg, Eg → Rul	Problem-based mixed approach.	A combination of problem-based and information-based learning.	Students have the option of an information orientated or problem-based approach.
7	Eg → Rul	Problem-initiated learning.	The problem is used as a trigger at the beginning of learning.	Patient management problems are used to interest the student in a topic.

Continued

	Terminology	Description	Example
8 Eg → Rul (Sp)	Problem-centred learning.	A study of the problem introduces the student to the principles and rules specific to the problem.	A text provides a series of problems followed by the information necessary to tackle the problems.
9 Eg — Rul (Sp)	Problem-centred discovery learning.	Following the presentation of the problem students have the opportunity to derive the principles and rules.	Students derive the principles from the literature or from work undertaken.
10 Eg — Rul (G)	Problem-based learning.	The development of the principles includes the generalisation stage of learning.	The investigation of patients with thyrotoxicosis is extended to a more general understanding of thyroid function tests.
11 Eg (T) — Rul	Task-based learning.	The problem is the real world.	A set of tasks undertaken by a health care professional are the basis for the 'problem' presented to the student.

APPENDIX 10

FOUR DIMENSIONS OF STUDENT PROGRESSION (reproduced with permission from Harden, 2007, Medical Teacher 29: 678–682.)

Increased Scope	
Increased Breadth	*Increased Difficulty*
A → A + B + C	A → A

• Extension to more or new topics
• Extension to different practice contexts
• Application of existing knowledge or skills to new knowledge or skills
	• More in-depth or advances consideration
	• Application to a more complex situation
	  – move from a uni-dimensional straightforward situation to one involving multiple problems or systems
	  – move to multifactorial problems involving different factors (eg, social, economical, medical)
	  – complications (eg, associated with treatment)
	• Less obvious or more subtle situations
	  – fewer cues
	  – less obvious cues
	  – atypical cues

Increased Utility	**Increased Proficiency**
Application (to medical practice)	*Increased Accomplishment*
A → A	A → A

• Move from general context to specific medical context
• Move from theory to practice of medicine
• Move to integration into the role of a doctor
  – an integrated repertoire involving a holistic approach to practice and bringing together the different abilities expected of a doctor
  – dealing with and reconciling competing demands, such as time spent on curative and preventive medicine
	• More efficient performance
	  – better organised
	  – more confident
	  – takes less time
	  – more accessible
	  – less unnecessary or redundant action
	  – higher standards
	  – lower errors
	• Less need for supervision
	• Takes initiative and anticipates events
	• Better able to defend and justify actions
	• Adapts routinely as part of practice

APPENDIX 11

FIRST TWO SECTIONS OF THE LEARNING OUTCOME/TASKS MASTERY GRID FOR VOCATIONAL TRAINING IN DENTISTRY (reproduced from Mitchell, Harden & Laidlaw, 1999, Medical Teacher 20: 91–98.)

	Tasks performed by the trainee*					
	Caries and restorations	Periodontal patient	Acute dental pain	Endodontic problem	Partial/complete denture	Minor surgical procedure
General						
Critically appraise and assess his or her own work	+	+	+	+	+	+
Keep up to date and continue with his or her education	+	+	+	+	+	+
Understand not only what he or she is doing, but why it is being done	+	+	+	+	+	+
Communication with patients						
History taking	+	+	+	+	+	+
Explanation of the clinical condition	+	+	+	+	+	+
Explanation of suggested treatment plan and alternatives	+	+	±	+	+	+
Explanation of cost and obtaining consent to pay	+	+	±	+	+	+
Explanation of preventive aspects of the patient's problem	+	+	+	+	−	+
Explanation of recognised complications related to treatment	+	−	−	+	+	+
Explanation of appliance inconvenience or failure	−	−	−	−	+	−
Explanation of necessary appliance	−	−	−	−	+	−

*applies +; may apply ±; does not apply −.

APPENDIX 12

DUNDEE READY EDUCATION ENVIRONMENT MEASURE (DREEM)
(reproduced with permission from McAleer and Roff, 2001, AMEE Guide
No. 23 Curriculum, Climate, Quality and Change in Medical Education:
A Unifying Perspective. Part 3 Appendix 1.)

Dundee Ready Education Measure (DREEM)

Age _____ Year of study _____ Male _____ Female _____

Medical School _____

Please indicate whether you:
Strongly Agree (SA), Agree (A), are Unsure (U), Disagree (D) or Strongly Disagree (SD) with the following
statements. Circle the appropriate response.

	SA	A	U	D	SD
1. I am encouraged to participate in class	SA	A	U	D	SD
2. The teachers are knowledgeable	SA	A	U	D	SD
3. There is a good support system for students who get stresses	SA	A	U	D	SD
4. I am too tired to enjoy the course	SA	A	U	D	SD
5. Learning strategies which worked for me before continue to work for me now	SA	A	U	D	SD
6. The teachers are patient with patients	SA	A	U	D	SD
7. The teaching is often stimulating	SA	A	U	D	SD
8. The teachers ridicule the students	SA	A	U	D	SD
9. The teachers are authoritarian	SA	A	U	D	SD
10. I am confident about my passing this year	SA	A	U	D	SD
11. The atmosphere is relaxed during the ward teaching	SA	A	U	D	SD
12. The school is well time tabled	SA	A	U	D	SD
13. The teaching is student centred	SA	A	U	D	SD
14. I am rarely bored on this course	SA	A	U	D	SD
15. I have good friends in this school	SA	A	U	D	SD
16. The teaching helps to develop my competence	SA	A	U	D	SD
17. Cheating is a problem in this school	SA	A	U	D	SD
18. The teachers have good communication skills with patients	SA	A	U	D	SD
19. My social life is good	SA	A	U	D	SD
20. The teaching is well focused	SA	A	U	D	SD
21. I feel I am being well prepared for my profession	SA	A	U	D	SD
22. The teaching helps to develop my confidence	SA	A	U	D	SD
23. The atmosphere is relaxed during lectures	SA	A	U	D	SD
24. The teaching time is put to good use	SA	A	U	D	SD
25. The teaching over-emphasises factual learning	SA	A	U	D	SD
26. Last year's work has been a good preparation for this year's work	SA	A	U	D	SD
27. I am able to memorise all I need	SA	A	U	D	SD
28. I seldom feel lonely	SA	A	U	D	SD
29. The teachers are good at providing feedback to students	SA	A	U	D	SD
30. There are opportunities for me to develop interpersonal skills	SA	A	U	D	SD
31. I have learned a lot about empathy in my profession	SA	A	U	D	SD
32. The teachers provide constructive criticism here	SA	A	U	D	SD
33. I feel comfortable in class socially	SA	A	U	D	SD
34. The atmosphere is relaxed during seminars/tutorials	SA	A	U	D	SD
35. I find the experience disappointing	SA	A	U	D	SD
36. I am able to concentrate well	SA	A	U	D	SD
37. The teachers give clear examples	SA	A	U	D	SD
38. I am clear about the learning objectives of the course	SA	A	U	D	SD
39. The teachers get angry in class	SA	A	U	D	SD
40. The teachers are well prepared for their classes	SA	A	U	D	SD
41. My problem solving skills are being well developed here	SA	A	U	D	SD
42. The enjoyment outweighs the stress of the course	SA	A	U	D	SD
43. The atmosphere motivates me as a learner	SA	A	U	D	SD
44. The teaching encourages me to be an active learner	SA	A	U	D	SD
45. Much of what I have to learn seems relevant to a career in healthcare	SA	A	U	D	SD
46. My accommodation is pleasant	SA	A	U	D	SD
47. Long term learning is emphasised over short term learning	SA	A	U	D	SD
48. The teaching to too teacher-centred	SA	A	U	D	SD
49. I feel able to ask the questions I want	SA	A	U	D	SD
50. The students irritate the teachers	SA	A	U	D	SD

APPENDIX 13

EVALUATION OF A LECTURE

Name of lecturer: _____

Date: _____

	Definitely yes	Probably yes	Uncertain	Probably no	Definitely no
1. The content of the lecture addressed the course learning outcomes	☐	☐	☐	☐	☐
2. The delivery of the lecture was clear and paced correctly	☐	☐	☐	☐	☐
3. Visual aids were used effectively	☐	☐	☐	☐	☐
4. I found the lecture stimulating	☐	☐	☐	☐	☐
5. The lecturer actively engaged students during the lecture	☐	☐	☐	☐	☐
6. Opportunities were provided to ask questions	☐	☐	☐	☐	☐
7. Useful handouts were provided	☐	☐	☐	☐	☐
8. The learning experience was valuable	☐	☐	☐	☐	☐
9. The lecture was pitched at the right level	☐	☐	☐	☐	☐
10. The lecturer kept to the time allocated	☐	☐	☐	☐	☐
11. The lecture was well prepared	☐	☐	☐	☐	☐

12. What did you most like about the lecture

13. What did you like least about the lecture

14. Any other comments

INDEX